MAKING SENSE OF THE ECG

To Kathryn and Caroline

MAKING SENSE OF THE ECG

A hands-on guide

Andrew R Houghton
MA(Oxon), BM BCh, MRCP(UK)
Cardiology Research Fellow & Honorary Registrar,
Department of Cardiovascular Medicine,
University Hospital, Queen's Medical Centre,
Nottingham, NG7 2UH, UK

David Gray
DM, MPH, BMedSci, BM BS, FRCP(UK)
Reader in Medicine & Honorary Consultant Physician,
Department of Cardiovascular Medicine,
University Hospital, Queen's Medical Centre,
Nottingham, NG7 2UH, UK

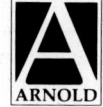

A member of the Hodder Headline Group
LONDON
Co-published in the USA by Oxford University Press, Inc., New York

First published in Great Britain in 1997 by
Arnold, a member of the Hodder Headline Group,
338 Euston Road, London NW1 3BH

Reprinted 1998 with updated material
Fourth impression 2001

Arnold International Students' Edition published 1998
Arnold International Student's Editions are low-priced un-abridged editions
of important textbooks. They are only for sale in developing countries.

Co-published in the United States of America by
Oxford University Press, Inc.,
198 Madison Avenue, New York, NY 10016
Oxford is a registered trademark of Oxford University Press

© 1997 A R Houghton and D Gray

All rights reserved. No part of this publication may be reproduced or
transmitted in any form or by any means, electronically or mechanically,
including photocopying, recording or any information storage or retrieval
system, without either prior permission in writing from the publisher or a
licence permitting restricted copying. In the United Kingdom such licences
are issued by the Copyright Licensing Agency: 90 Tottenham Court Road,
London WIP 9HE.

Whilst the advice and information in this book is believed to be true and
accurate at the date of going to press, neither the authors nor the publisher
can accept any legal responsibility or liability for any errors or omissions
that may be made. In particular (but without limiting the generality of the
preceding disclaimer) every effort has been made to check drug dosages;
however, it is still possible that errors have been missed. Furthermore,
dosage schedules are constantly being revised and new side-effects
recognized. For these reasons the reader is strongly urged to consult the
drug companies' printed instructions before administering any of the drugs
recommended in this book.

British Library Cataloguing in Publication Data
A catalogue record for this book is available from the British Library

Library of Congress Cataloging-in-Publication Data
A catalog record for this book is available from the Library of Congress

ISBN 0 340 70100 5

Composition by Scribe Design, Gillingham, Kent, UK
Printed and bound in India by Ajanta Offset

Winner of two academic medical prizes:
Royal Society of Medicine 1997 and British Medical Association 1998

This book has now been translated into the following languages:
Spanish, Italian, Japanese, Chinese, Polish, Turkish, Hungarian
and Russian

CONTENTS

Where to find the ECGs	vi
Where to find the medical conditions	xiii
Preface	xvii
Acknowledgements	xix
1 PQRST: where the waves come from	1
2 Heart rate	21
3 Rhythm	31
4 The axis	77
5 The P wave	97
6 The PR interval	109
7 The Q wave	125
8 The QRS complex	133
9 The ST segment	155
10 The T wave	179
11 The QT interval	195
12 The U wave	207
13 Artefacts on the ECG	213
14 Pacemakers	219
15 Exercise ECG testing	227
16 Cardiopulmonary resuscitation	239
Further reading	255
Help with the next edition	257
Index	259

WHERE TO FIND THE ECGS

ECG and Figure number	Page number

Accelerated idioventricular rhythm
3.20 58
Anterior myocardial infarction
7.4, 9.5, 10.3 .... 129, 161, 183
Asystole
16.3 244
Atrial ectopics
3.25 63
Atrial fibrillation
3.13, 5.2 .... 45, 99
Atrial flutter (3:1 AV block)
3.11 43
Atrial tachycardia
3.9 41
AV block, 2:1
6.10 120
AV block, first degree
6.7 116
AV block, Mobitz type I
6.8 118
AV block, Mobitz type II
6.9 119
AV block, third-degree
3.31, 6.11 .... 70, 121
AV dissociation
3.32 70
AV junctional ectopics
3.26 64
AV junctional escape rhythm
3.23 62
AV junctional tachycardia
5.4, 5.7 .... 101, 104
AV nodal re-entry tachycardia
3.17 51
AV re-entry tachycardia (WPW syndrome)
3.16 50

Bifascicular block
4.17 91
Bigeminy
3.28 65
Bundle branch block, incomplete left
8.17 152
Bundle branch block, incomplete right
8.18 153
Bundle branch block, left
8.11 146
Bundle branch block, right
8.15 149

Capture beats
3.37 75
Carotid sinus massage
3.12 44
Complete AV block
3.31, 6.11 .... 70, 121

Delta wave (WPW syndrome)
6.4, 6.5 .... 112, 113
Dextrocardia
8.5 140
Digoxin effect
9.14 175
Digoxin toxicity
10.9 193
Dual-chamber sequential pacing
14.2 225

Ectopic beats, atrial
3.25 63
Ectopic beats, AV junctional
3.26 64
Ectopic beats, bigeminy
3.28 65
Ectopic beats, ventricular
3.27, 3.34, 8.16 .... 65, 72, 150
Electrical alternans
8.7 143

Electrode misplacement
13.1 214
Electromechanical dissociation
16.4 244
Exercise test (coronary artery disease)
15.3 235

First-degree AV block
6.7 116
Fusion beats
3.36 74

High take-off
9.12 170
Hypercalcaemia
11.2 198
Hyperkalaemia
10.2 181
Hypertrophy, left ventricular
7.6, 8.2. . . . . 132, 136
Hypertrophy, left ventricular with strain
9.15 177
Hypertrophy, right ventricular with strain
8.3 137
Hypocalcaemia
11.3 202
Hypokalaemia
10.4, 12.2 . . . . 185, 209

Incomplete left bundle branch block
8.17 152
Incomplete right bundle branch block
8.18 153
Incorrect calibration
13.3 216
Incorrect paper speed
13.4 217
Inferior myocardial infarction
1.9, 7.5, 9.6. . . . . 8, 130, 162

J point
15.2 232

Lateral myocardial infarction
  1.10, 9.4. . . . . 9, 160
Left axis deviation
  4.16 90
Left bundle branch block
  8.11 146
Left bundle branch block, incomplete
  8.17 152
Left ventricular aneurysm
  9.9 165
Left ventricular hypertrophy
  7.6, 8.2. . . . . 132, 136
Left ventricular hypertrophy with strain
  9.15 177
Long QT interval
  11.3 202
Lown–Ganong–Levine syndrome
  6.6 114

Mobitz type I AV block
  6.8 118
Mobitz type II AV block
  6.9 119
Myocardial infarction, anterior
  7.4, 9.5, 10.3 . . . . 129, 161, 183
Myocardial infarction, inferior
  1.9, 7.5, 9.6. . . . . 8, 130, 162
Myocardial infarction, lateral
  1.10, 9.4. . . . . 9, 160
Myocardial infarction, non-Q wave
  10.8 191
Myocardial infarction, posterior
  8.4 138
Myocardial infarction, Q wave
  10.7 190
Myocardial infarction, right ventricular
  9.8 163
Myocardial ischaemia
  9.13, 10.6, 15.3. . . . . 172, 189, 235

Non-Q wave myocardial infarction
  10.8 191

Normal 12-lead ECG
8.1, 10.1 .... 133, 180
Normal T wave inversion
10.5 187

P mitrale
5.9 107
P pulmonale
5.8 105
Pacing – dual-chamber sequential
14.2 225
Pacing – ventricular
14.1 224
Pericardial effusion
8.6, 8.7 .... 142, 143
Pericarditis
9.11 168
Posterior myocardial infarction
8.4 138
Prinzmetal's angina
9.10 168
Q wave myocardial infarction
10.7 190
Q wave, normal
7.3 127
QT interval, long
11.3 202
QT interval, short
11.2 198

Right axis deviation
4.19 94
Right bundle branch block
8.15 149
Right bundle branch block, incomplete
8.18 153
Right ventricular hypertrophy with strain
8.3 137
Right ventricular myocardial infarction
9.8 163

Short QT interval
11.2 198
Signal-averaged ECG
13.5 218
Sinoatrial block
3.7, 3.33....................................... 39, 72
Sinus arrest
3.6, 5.3.. 38, 100
Sinus arrhythmia
3.5 37
Sinus bradycardia
3.3 34
Sinus rhythm
3.2, 5.1 .... 33, 98
Sinus tachycardia
3.4, 5.5.. 36, 102

T wave inversion (normal)
10.5 187
Tachycardia, AV junctional
5.4, 5.7....................................... 101, 104
Tachycardia, sinus
3.4, 5.5....................................... 36, 102
Tachycardia, ventricular
3.19, 3.35, 3.36, 3.37, 16.2.................. 55, 74, 75, 243
Tense patient
1.1... 2
Third-degree AV block
3.31, 6.11..................................... 70, 121
Torsades de pointes
3.21 58
Trifascicular block
4.18 92

U wave
12.1, 12.2..................................... 207, 209

Vasospastic angina
9.10 167
Ventricular ectopics
3.27, 3.34, 8.16 .... 65, 72, 150

Ventricular escape rhythm
3.24 62
Ventricular fibrillation
3.19, 16.1 .... 55, 243
Ventricular pacing
14.1 224
Ventricular tachycardia
3.19, 3.35, 3.36, 3.37, 16.2 .... 55, 74, 75, 243

Wolff–Parkinson–White syndrome
6.4, 6.5 .... 112, 113

WHERE TO FIND THE MEDICAL CONDITIONS

Medical condition	Page number

Abnormal atrial depolarization 104
Accelerated idioventricular rhythm 57
Anterolateral myocardial infarction 160
Asystole 25, 244
Atrial enlargement, left 106
Atrial enlargement, right 105–106
Atrial fibrillation 44–48
Atrial flutter 42–44
Atrial tachycardia 40–42
AV block, 2:1 . . . . 117, 120
AV block, first-degree 60, 90, 115–116
AV block, Mobitz type I 117–118
AV block, Mobitz type II 117, 119–120
AV block, third-degree 24, 60, 90, 117–118, 121–122
AV dissociation 70, 71, 122
AV junctional rhythms 69
AV re-entry tachycardia 48–54

Bradycardia 23, 24–26, 30
Bundle branch block 60–61, 144–150

Complete heart block 24, 60, 90, 117–118, 121–122
Conduction disturbances 60–61

Dextrocardia 139–140
Digoxin 174–175
Digoxin toxicity 41, 174–175

Ectopic beats 63–66, 71
Electromechanical dissociation 244
Escape rhythms 25, 35, 61–63

Fascicular block 152–153
First-degree AV block 60, 90, 115–116

Hemiblock, left anterior..............................89–91
Hemiblock, left posterior..............................95
Hereditary long-QT syndromes......................59, 205
High take-off....................................170–171
Hypercalcaemia.............................198–200, 210
Hyperkalaemia...............................181–182
Hyperthyroidism....................................210
Hypertrophy, left ventricular....................131, 135, 192
Hypertrophy, right ventricular................93, 136–137, 192
Hypocalcaemia..................................201–203
Hypokalaemia..........................184–185, 209–210
Hypothyroidism....................................186

Incomplete bundle branch block.....................151–152
Inferior myocardial infarction................6–8, 160, 161, 162

Left anterior hemiblock..............................89–91
Left atrial enlargement...............................106
Left posterior hemiblock..............................95
Left ventricular aneurysm..........................165–166
Left ventricular hypertrophy....................131, 135, 192
Lown–Ganong–Levine syndrome.....................114–115

Mobitz type I AV block............................117–118
Mobitz type II AV block........................117, 119–120
Myocardial infarction..............................156–164
Myocardial infarction, anterolateral......................160
Myocardial infarction, inferior...............6–8, 160, 161, 162
Myocardial infarction, posterior........................173
Myocardial infarction, right ventricular................163–164
Myocardial ischaemia.............................171–173
Myocarditis..203

Pacemakers and surgery...........................225–226
Pericardial effusion............................141–143, 186
Pericarditis....................................169–170
Posterior myocardial infarction........................173
Prinzmetal's angina...............................166–168
Pulseless ventricular tachycardia........................243

Right atrial enlargement...........................105–106

Right ventricular hypertrophy................... 93, 136–137, 192
Right ventricular myocardial infarction.................. 163–164

Sick sinus syndrome............................. 24, 38–40
Sinus arrhythmia................................ 37–38, 98
Sinus bradycardia........................... 24, 25, 34–35
Sinus rhythm... 32–34
Sinus tachycardia..................................... 35–37
Surgery and pacemakers............................. 225–226

Tachycardia................................. 23, 27–29, 30
Third-degree AV block.............. 24, 60, 90, 117–118, 121–122
Torsades de pointes........................... 57–59, 203, 205

Unstable angina...................................... 173

Vasospastic angina................................ 166–168
Ventricular fibrillation....................... 28, 55, 59, 243
Ventricular hypertrophy............... 93, 131, 135, 136–137, 192
Ventricular hypertrophy with strain............... 176, 177, 192
Ventricular rhythms........................ 67–68, 76, 151
Ventricular tachycardia............................... 55–59
Ventricular tachycardia, pulseless....................... 243

Wolff–Parkinson–White syndrome.................... 111–114

PREFACE

Whether you are a physician, surgeon, general practitioner, nurse, paramedic or medical student, you will have to assess ECGs at some point in your career. This book is written to help you do just that.

The aim of this book is to guide you through the recognition and interpretation of ECG abnormalities. It is not sufficient, however, simply to know what is wrong with an ECG. You also need to know what to do about it, so the book will help you to decide whether abnormalities are significant or not and, most important of all, when you should ask for help.

Although this book will help you to interpret ECGs, it cannot be overemphasized that this should always be done in combination with a thorough assessment of the patient. The ECG is undoubtedly a valuable tool, but only when combined with a detailed patient history and physical examination.

Andrew R Houghton
David Gray
Nottingham, June 1996

ACKNOWLEDGEMENTS

We would like to thank everyone who gave us suggestions and constructive criticism while we prepared this book. We are particularly grateful to Ian Ferrer, Michael Holmes, Safiy Karim, Dave Kendall, Martin Melville, Neville Smith and Gary Spiers for providing us with their invaluable comments on the final draft of the text. We are also indebted to Iain Lyburn and Sonia Magnago for allowing us to use ECGs from their collections, and to everyone at Arnold for their guidance and support.

PQRST: WHERE THE WAVES COME FROM

The electrocardiogram (ECG) is one of the most widely used and useful investigations in contemporary medicine. It is essential for the identification of disorders of the cardiac rhythm, extremely useful for the diagnosis of abnormalities of the heart (such as myocardial infarction), and a helpful clue to the presence of generalized disorders that affect the rest of the body too (such as electrolyte disturbances).

Each chapter in this book will consider a specific feature of the ECG in turn. We begin, however, with an overview of the ECG in which we will explain the following points:

- What does the ECG actually record?
- How does the ECG 'look' at the heart?
- What do the waves mean?
- How do I record an ECG?

We recommend you take some time to read through this chapter before trying to interpret ECG abnormalities. For an excellent and more detailed primer on the ECG, we recommend J. R. Hampton's *The ECG Made Easy*.

2 MAKING SENSE OF THE ECG

What does the ECG actually record?

ECG machines record the electrical activity of the heart. They also pick up the activity of other muscles, such as skeletal muscle. ECG machines are designed to filter this out as much as possible, but encouraging patients to relax during an ECG recording helps to obtain a clear trace (Fig. 1.1).

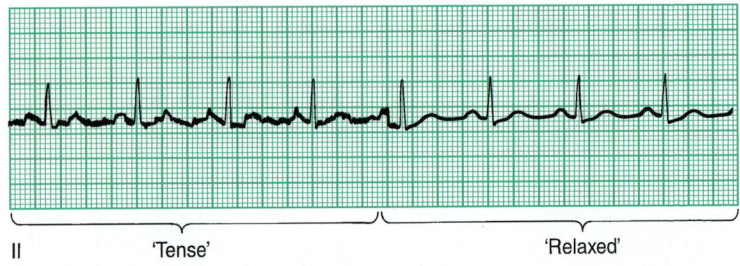

FIG. 1.1

An ECG from a relaxed patient is much easier to interpret

Key points:
- electrical interference (irregular baseline) when patient is tense
- clearer recording when patient relaxes

By convention, the main waves on the ECG are given the names P, Q, R, S, T and U (Fig. 1.2). Each wave represents depolarization ('electrical discharging') or repolarization ('electrical recharging') of a certain region of the heart – this is discussed in more detail in the rest of this chapter.

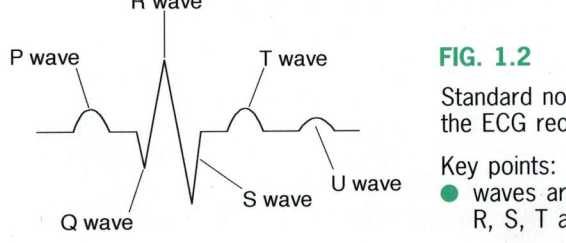

FIG. 1.2

Standard nomenclature of the ECG recording

Key points:
- waves are called P, Q, R, S, T and U

PQRST: WHERE THE WAVES COME FROM

The voltage changes detected by ECG machines are very small, being of the order of millivolts. The size of each wave corresponds to the amount of voltage generated by the event which created it: the greater the voltage, the larger the wave (Fig. 1.3).

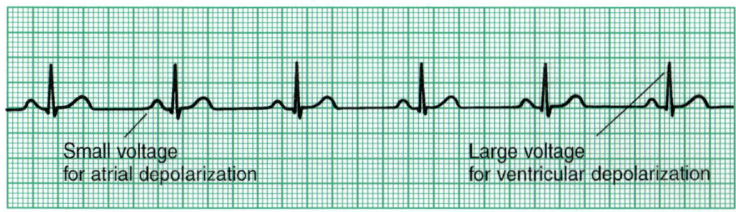

II

FIG. 1.3
The size of a wave reflects the voltage that caused it

Key points:
- P waves are small (atrial depolarization generates little voltage)
- QRS complexes are larger (ventricular depolarization generates a higher voltage)

The ECG also allows you to calculate how long an event lasted. The ECG paper moves through the machine at a constant rate of 25 mm/s, so by measuring the width of a P wave, for example, you can calculate the duration of atrial depolarization (Fig. 1.4).

How does the ECG 'look' at the heart?

To make sense of the ECG, one of the most important concepts to understand is that of the 'lead'. This is a term you will often see, and it does **not** refer to the wires that connect the patient to the ECG machine (which we will always refer to as 'electrodes' to avoid confusion).

In short, 'leads' are different viewpoints of the heart's electrical activity. An ECG machine uses the information it

4 MAKING SENSE OF THE ECG

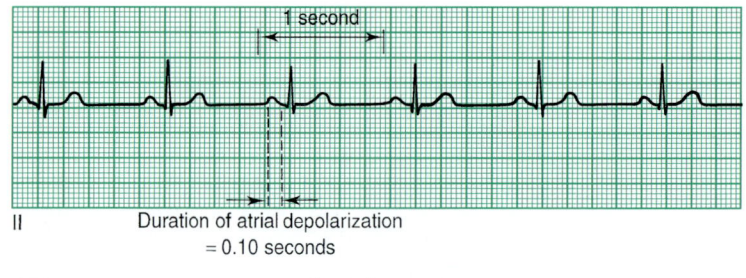

II   Duration of atrial depolarization = 0.10 seconds

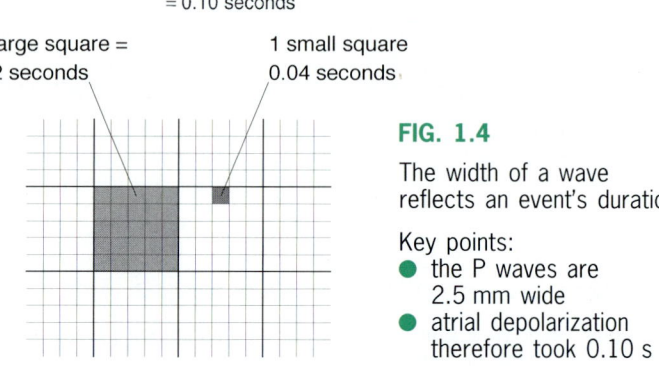

FIG. 1.4

The width of a wave reflects an event's duration

Key points:
- the P waves are 2.5 mm wide
- atrial depolarization therefore took 0.10 s

collects via its four limb and six chest electrodes to compile a comprehensive picture of the electrical activity in the heart as observed from 12 different viewpoints, and this set of 12 views or leads gives the 12-lead ECG its name.

Each lead is given a name (I, II, III, aVR, aVL, aVF, V_1, V_2, V_3, V_4, V_5 and V_6) and its position on a 12-lead ECG is usually standardized to make pattern recognition easier.

So what viewpoint does each lead have of the heart? Information from the four limb electrodes is used by the ECG machine to create the six limb leads (I, II, III, aVR, aVL and aVF). Each limb lead 'looks' at the heart from the side (the coronal plane), and the angle at which it looks at the heart in this plane depends upon the lead in question (Fig. 1.5). Thus, lead aVR looks at the heart from the approximate viewpoint of the patient's right shoulder, whereas lead aVL looks from the left shoulder and lead aVF looks directly upward from the feet.

PQRST: WHERE THE WAVES COME FROM

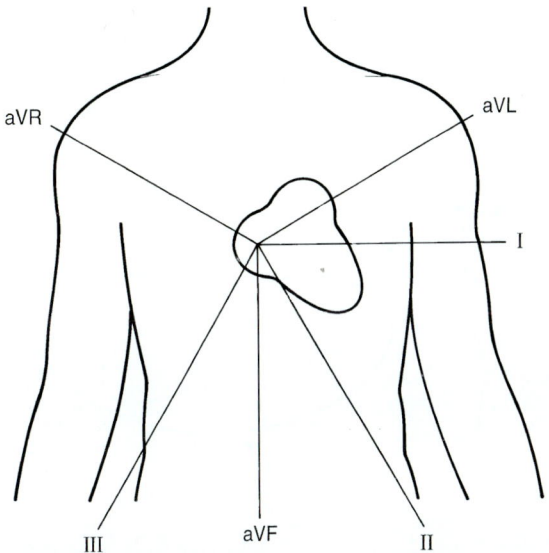

FIG. 1.5

The viewpoint each limb lead has of the heart

Key points:
- each limb lead looks at the heart in the coronal plane
- each lead looks at the heart from a different angle

The six chest leads (V_1 to V_6) look at the heart in a horizontal plane from the front and around the side of the chest (Fig. 1.6).

The region of myocardium surveyed by each lead therefore varies according to its vantage point – lead aVF has a good 'view' of the inferior surface of the heart, and lead V_3 has a good view of the anterior surface, for example.

Once you know the view each lead has of the heart, you can tell if the electrical impulses in the heart are flowing towards that lead or away from it. This is very simple to work out, because electrical current flowing towards a lead produces an upward (positive) deflection on the ECG,

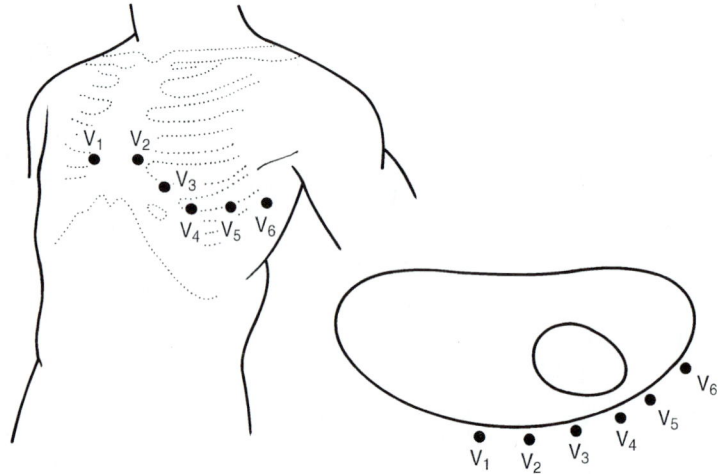

FIG. 1.6

The viewpoint each chest lead has of the heart

Key points:
- each chest lead looks at the heart in the transverse plane
- each lead looks at the heart from a different angle

whereas current flowing away causes a downward (negative) deflection (Fig. 1.7).

We will discuss the origin of each wave shortly, but just as an example consider the P wave, which represents atrial depolarization. The P wave is positive in lead II because atrial depolarization flows towards that lead, but it is negative in lead aVR because this looks at the atria from the opposite direction (Fig. 1.8).

In addition to working out the direction of flow of electrical current, knowing the viewpoint of each lead allows you to determine which regions of the heart are affected by, for example, myocardial infarction. Infarction of the inferior surface will produce changes in the leads looking at that

PQRST: WHERE THE WAVES COME FROM 7

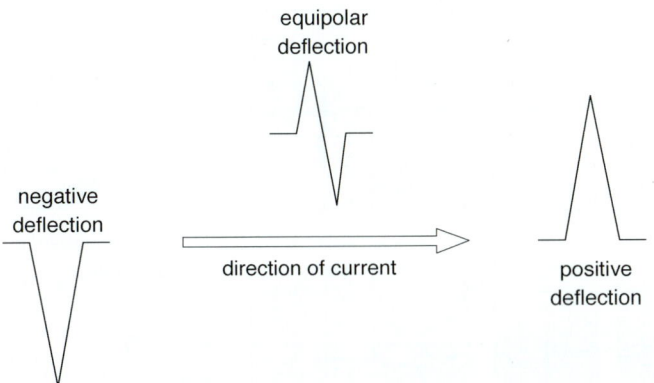

FIG. 1.7

The direction of an ECG deflection depends upon the direction of the current

Key points:
- flow towards a lead produces a positive deflection
- flow away from a lead produces a negative deflection
- flow past a lead produces a positive then a negative (equipolar) deflection

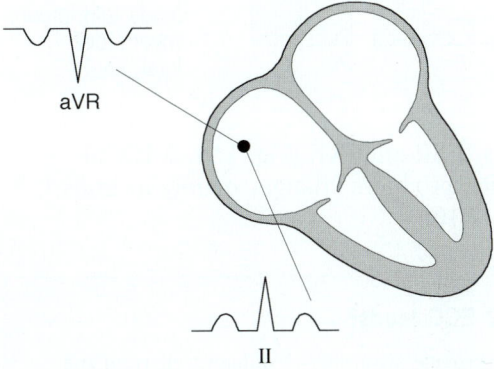

FIG. 1.8

The orientation of the P wave depends upon the lead

Key points:
- P waves are normally upright in lead II
- P waves are normally inverted in lead aVR

8 MAKING SENSE OF THE ECG

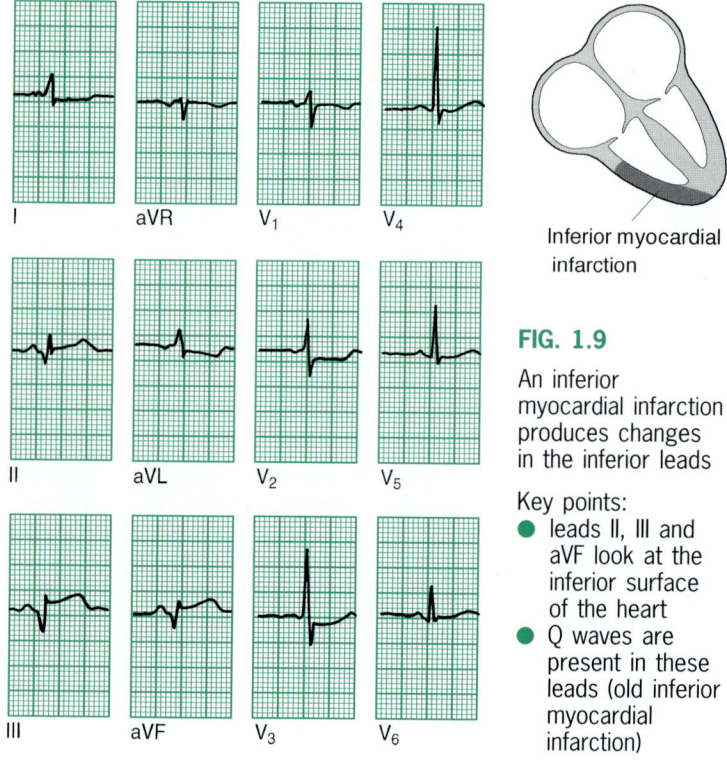

Inferior myocardial infarction

FIG. 1.9

An inferior myocardial infarction produces changes in the inferior leads

Key points:
- leads II, III and aVF look at the inferior surface of the heart
- Q waves are present in these leads (old inferior myocardial infarction)

region, namely leads II, III and aVF (Fig. 1.9). A lateral infarction, meanwhile, produces changes mainly in leads I, aVL, V$_5$ and V$_6$ (Fig. 1.10).

Why are there 12 ECG leads?

Twelve leads simply provide a number of different views of the heart that are manageable (too many leads would take too long to interpret) yet provide a comprehensive picture of the heart's electrical activity (too few leads might 'overlook' important regions). For research purposes, where a more detailed picture of the heart is needed, over 100 leads are often used.

PQRST: WHERE THE WAVES COME FROM

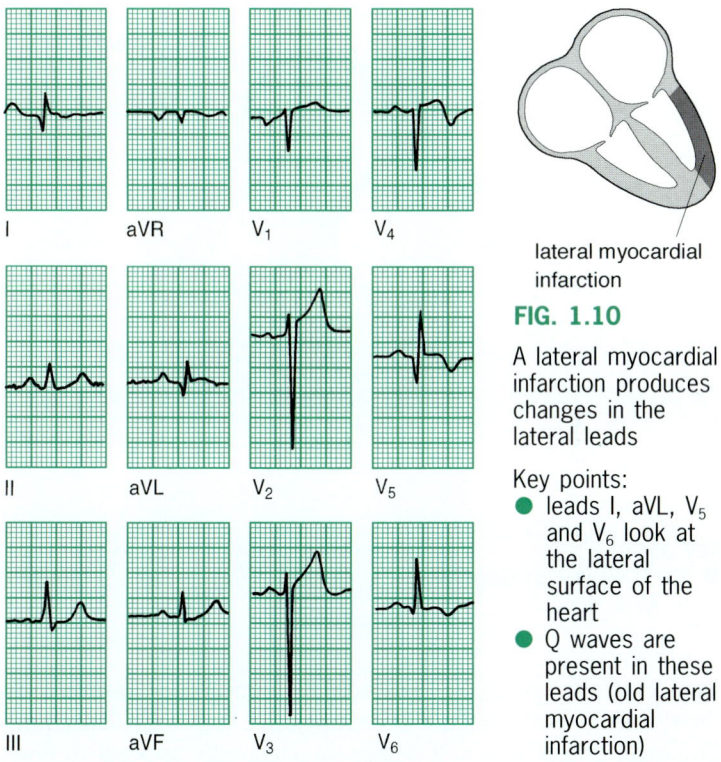

lateral myocardial infarction

FIG. 1.10

A lateral myocardial infarction produces changes in the lateral leads

Key points:
- leads I, aVL, V$_5$ and V$_6$ look at the lateral surface of the heart
- Q waves are present in these leads (old lateral myocardial infarction)

Where do the waves come from?

In the normal heart, each beat begins with the discharge ('depolarization') of the sinoatrial (SA) node, high up in the right atrium. This is a spontaneous event, occurring 60–100 times every minute.

Depolarization of the SA node does not cause any noticeable wave on the ECG. The first detectable wave appears when the impulse spreads from the SA node to depolarize the atria (Fig. 1.11). This produces the **P wave**.

The atria contain relatively little muscle, and so the voltage generated by atrial depolarization is relatively small. From the

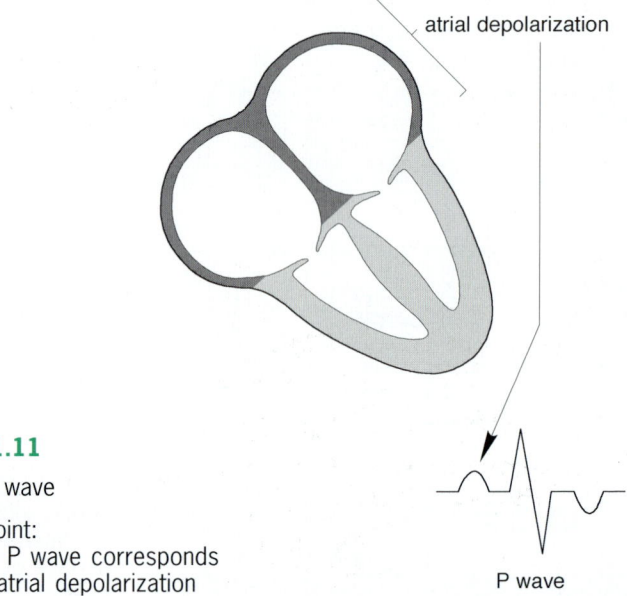

FIG. 1.11

The P wave

Key point:
- the P wave corresponds to atrial depolarization

viewpoint of most leads, the electricity appears to flow *towards* them and so the P wave will be a positive (upward) deflection. The exception is lead aVR where the electricity appears to flow *away* and so the P wave is negative in that lead (Fig. 1.8).

After flowing through the atria, the electrical impulse reaches the atrioventricular (AV) node, located low in the right atrium. The AV node is normally the only route by which an electrical impulse can reach the ventricles, the rest of the atrial myocardium being separated from the ventricles by a non-conducting ring of fibrous tissue.

Activation of the AV node does not produce an obvious wave on the ECG, but it does contribute to the time interval between the P wave and the subsequent Q or R wave. It does this by delaying conduction, and in doing so acts as a safety mechanism, preventing rapid atrial impulses from spreading to the ventricles at the same rate.

The time taken for the depolarization wave to pass from its origin in the SA node, across the atria, and through the AV node into ventricular muscle is called the **PR interval**. This is measured from the beginning of the P wave to the beginning of the R wave, and is normally between 0.12 and 0.20 s, or 3–5 small squares (Fig. 1.12).

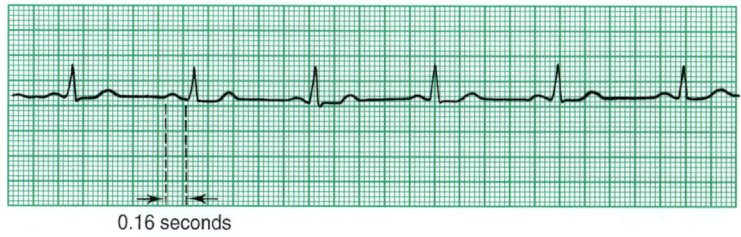

0.16 seconds

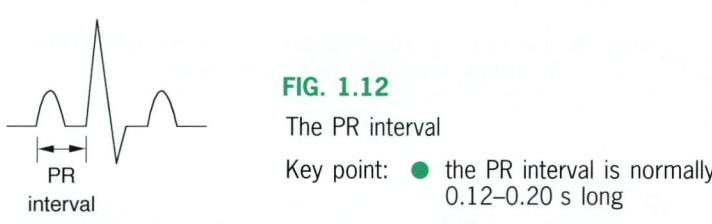

PR interval

FIG. 1.12

The PR interval

Key point: ● the PR interval is normally 0.12–0.20 s long

Once the impulse has traversed the AV node, it enters the bundle of His, a specialized conducting pathway which passes into the interventricular septum and divides into the left and right bundle branches (Fig. 1.13).

Current normally flows between the bundle branches in the interventricular septum, from left to right, and this is responsible for the first deflection of the **QRS complex**. Whether this is a downward deflection or an upward deflection depends upon which side of the septum a lead is 'looking' from (Fig. 1.14).

By convention, if the first deflection of the QRS complex is downward, it is called a **Q wave**. The first upward deflection is called an **R wave**, whether or not it follows a Q wave. A

12 MAKING SENSE OF THE ECG

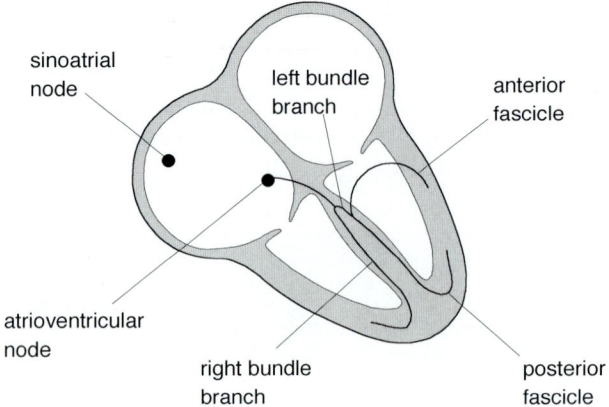

FIG. 1.13

The right and left bundle branches

Key points: ● the bundle of His divides into right and left bundle branches in the interventricular septum

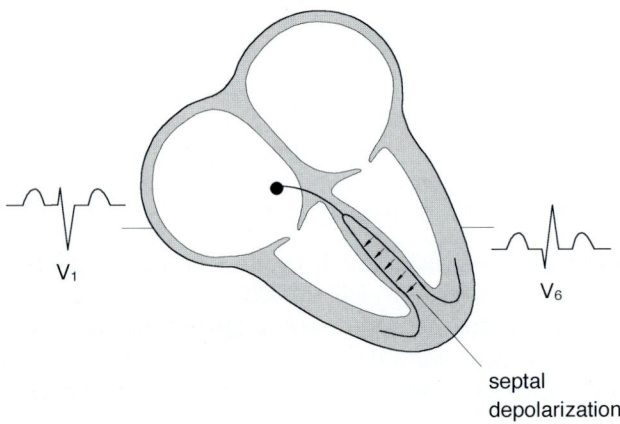

FIG. 1.14

Septal depolarization

Key point: ● the septum normally depolarizes from left to right

PQRST: WHERE THE WAVES COME FROM

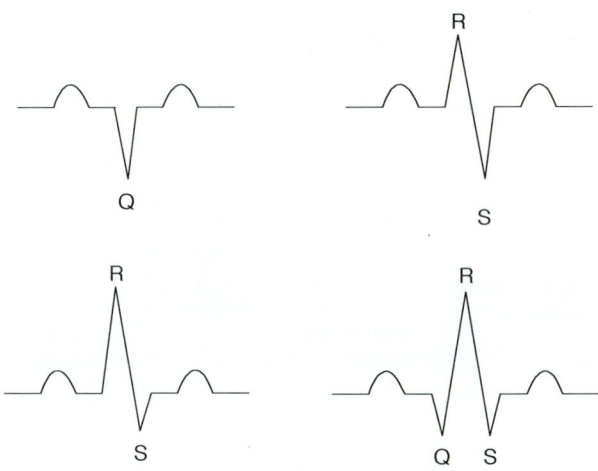

FIG. 1.15

The different varieties of QRS complex

Key points:
- the first downward deflection is a Q wave
- the first upward deflection is an R wave
- a downward deflection after an R wave is an S wave

downward deflection after an R wave is called an **S wave**. Hence, a variety of complexes are possible (Fig. 1.15).

The right bundle branch conducts the wave of depolarization to the right ventricle, whereas the left bundle branch divides into anterior and posterior fascicles which conduct the wave to the left ventricle (Fig. 1.16). The conducting pathways end by dividing into Purkinje fibres which distribute the wave of depolarization rapidly throughout both ventricles. The depolarization of the ventricles, represented by the QRS complex, is normally complete within 0.12 s (Fig. 1.17).

QRS complexes are 'positive' or 'negative' depending on whether the R wave or the S wave is bigger (Fig. 1.18). This, in turn, will depend upon the view each lead has of the heart.

14 MAKING SENSE OF THE ECG

FIG. 1.16

Divisions of the left bundle branch

Key point:
- the left bundle branch divides into anterior and posterior fascicles

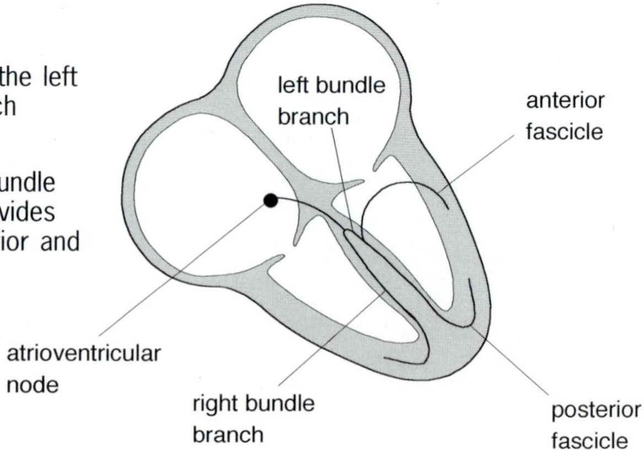

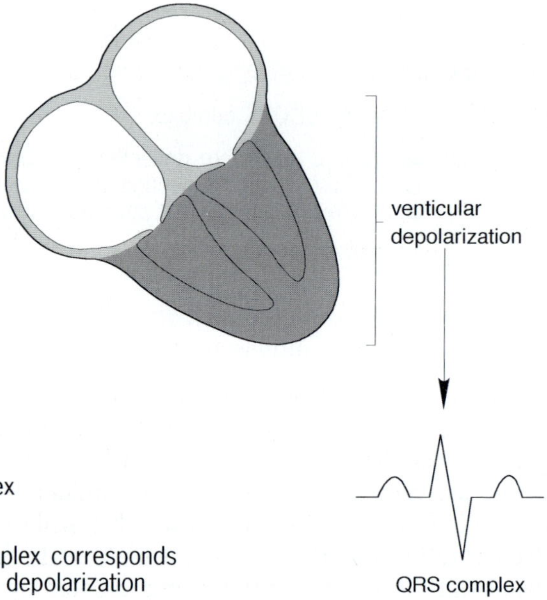

FIG. 1.17

The QRS complex

Key point:
- the QRS complex corresponds to ventricular depolarization

The left ventricle contains considerably more myocardium than the right, and so the voltage generated by its depolarization will tend to dominate the shape of the QRS complex.

PQRST: WHERE THE WAVES COME FROM

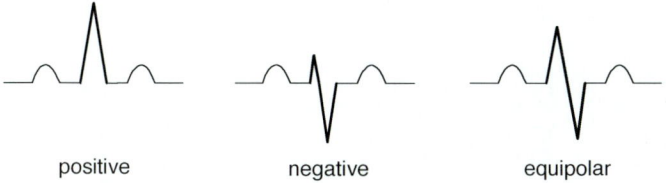

FIG. 1.18

Polarity of the QRS complexes

Key points:
- a dominant R wave means a positive QRS complex
- a dominant S wave means a negative QRS complex
- equal R and S waves mean an equipolar QRS complex

Leads that look at the heart from the right will see a relatively small amount of voltage moving towards them as the right ventricle depolarizes, and a larger amount moving away with depolarization of the left. The QRS complex will therefore be dominated by an S wave, and be negative. Conversely, leads looking at the heart from the left will see a relatively large voltage moving towards them, and a smaller voltage moving away, giving rise to a large R wave and only a small S wave (Fig. 1.19). Therefore, there is a gradual transition across the

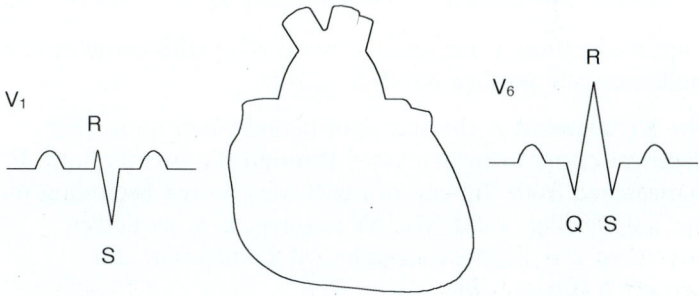

FIG. 1.19

QRS-complex shape varies according to the lead's viewpoint

Key points:
- right-sided leads have negative QRS complexes
- left-sided leads have positive QRS complexes

16 MAKING SENSE OF THE ECG

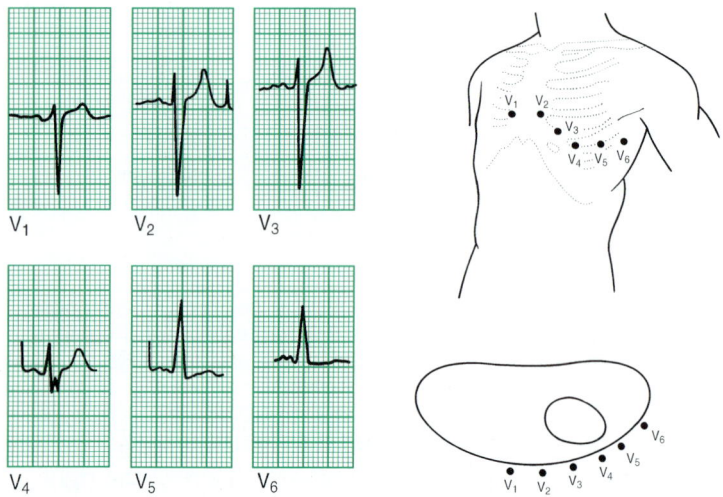

FIGURE 1.20

Transition in QRS complexes across the chest leads

Key points:
- QRS complexes are normally negative in leads V_1 and V_2
- QRS complexes are normally positive in leads V_5 and V_6

chest leads, from a predominantly negative QRS complex to a predominantly positive one (Fig. 1.20).

The **ST segment** is the transient period when no further electrical current can be passed through the myocardium. It is measured from the end of the S wave to the beginning of the T wave (Fig. 1.21). The ST segment is of particular interest in the diagnosis of myocardial infarction and ischaemia (Chapter 9).

The **T wave** represents repolarization ('recharging') of the ventricular myocardium to its resting electrical state. The **QT interval** measures the total time for activation of the ventricles and recovery to the normal resting state (Fig. 1.22).

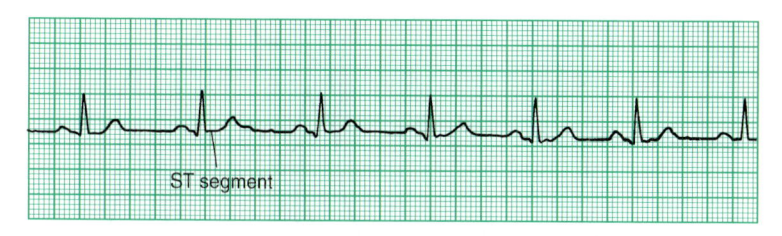

FIG. 1.21
The ST segment

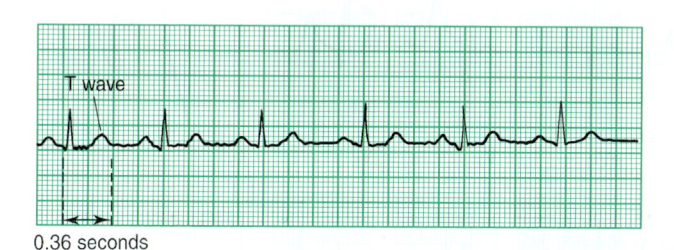

FIG. 1.22
The T wave and QT interval

0.36 seconds

The origin of the **U wave** is uncertain, but it may represent repolarization of the interventricular septum or slow repolarization of the ventricles. U waves can be difficult to identify but, when present, they are most clearly seen in the anterior chest leads V_2–V_4 (Fig. 1.23).

You need to be familiar with the most important electrical events which make up the cardiac cycle. These are summarized at the end of the chapter.

How do I record an ECG?

Always ensure you know how to operate the ECG machine before attempting to record an ECG. An incorrect recording can lead to incorrect diagnoses, wasted investigations and potentially disastrous unnecessary treatment.

Summary

The waves and intervals of the ECG correspond to the following events:

ECG event	Cardiac event
P wave	Atrial depolarization
PR interval	Start of atrial depolarization to start of ventricular depolarization
QRS complex	Ventricular depolarization
ST segment	Pause in ventricular electrical activity before repolarization
T wave	Ventricular repolarization
QT interval	Total time taken by ventricular depolarization and repolarization
U wave	Uncertain. Possibly:

- interventricular septal repolarization
- slow ventricular repolarization

Note: Depolarization of the SA and AV nodes are important events but do not *in themselves* produce a detectable wave on the standard ECG.

2

HEART RATE

Measurement of the heart rate and the identification of the cardiac rhythm go hand in hand, as many abnormalities of heart rate result from arrhythmias. How to identify the cardiac rhythm is discussed in detail in the following chapter. To begin with, however, we will simply describe ways to measure the heart rate and the abnormalities that can affect it.

When we talk of measuring the heart rate, we usually mean the *ventricular* rate, which corresponds to the patient's pulse. Depolarization of the ventricles produces the QRS complex on the ECG, and so it is the rate of QRS complexes that we want to measure to determine the heart rate.

Measurement of the heart rate is simple and can be done in several ways. Before you try and measure anything, however, check that the ECG has been recorded at the standard UK and USA paper speed of 25 mm/s. If so, then all you have to remember is that a 1-min ECG tracing covers **300 large squares**. If the patient's rhythm is regular, all you have to do is count the number of large squares between two QRS complexes, and divide it into 300. For example, in Fig. 2.1 there are 5 large squares between each QRS complex. Therefore:

$$\text{Heart rate} = \frac{300}{5} = 60 \text{ per minute}$$

22 MAKING SENSE OF THE ECG

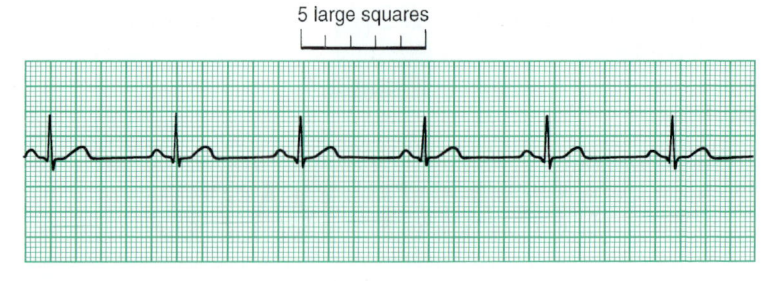

FIG. 2.1

Calculating heart rate when the rhythm is regular

Key points:
- 1 QRS complex every 5 large squares
- 300 large squares correspond to 1 min

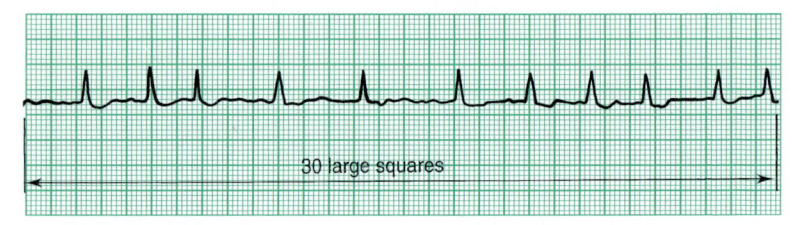

FIG. 2.2

Calculating heart rate when the rhythm is irregular

Key points:
- 30 large squares contain 11 QRS complexes
- 30 large squares correspond to 6 s

This method does not work so well when the rhythm is irregular, as the number of large squares between each QRS complex varies from beat to beat. Instead, count the number of QRS complexes in 30 large squares (Fig. 2.2). This is the number of QRS complexes in 6 s. To work out the rate per minute, simply multiply by 10:

Number of QRS complexes in 30 squares = 11
Number of QRS complexes in 6 s = 11
Therefore, number of QRS complexes per minute = 11 × 10
= 110

HEART RATE

An ECG ruler can be helpful, but follow the instructions on it carefully. Some ECG machines will calculate heart rate and print it on the ECG, but always check machine-derived values as machines do occasionally make errors!

Whichever method you use, remember they can be used to measure the atrial or P wave rate as well as the ventricular or QRS rate. Normally, every P wave is followed by a QRS complex and so the atrial and ventricular rates are the same. However, the rates can be different if, for example, some or all of the P waves are prevented from activating the ventricles (Fig. 2.3). Situations where this may happen are described in later chapters.

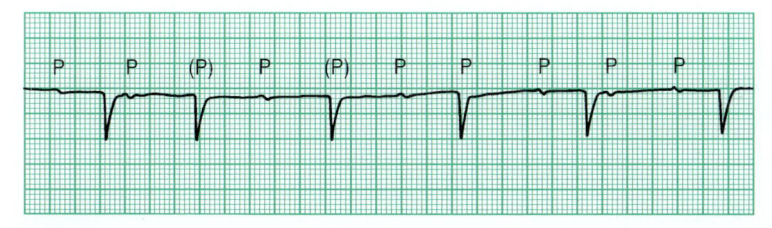

FIG. 2.3

The P wave rate can differ from the QRS complex rate

Key points:
- P wave (atrial) rate is 105 per minute
- QRS complex (ventricular) rate is 60 per minute

Once you have measured the heart rate, you need to decide whether it is normal or abnormal. As a general rule, a regular heart rhythm with a rate between 60 and 100 beats per minute is normal. If the rate is below 60 beats per minute, the patient is said to be **bradycardic**. With a heart rate above 100 beats per minute, the patient is **tachycardic**. Therefore, the two questions you need to ask about heart rate are:

- Is the heart rate below 60 beats per minute?
- Is the heart rate above 100 beats per minute?

If the answer to either question is 'yes', turn to the appropriate half of this chapter to find out what to do next. If not, turn to Chapter 3 to identify the cardiac rhythm.

IS THE HEART RATE BELOW 60 BEATS PER MINUTE?

Bradycardia is arbitrarily defined as a heart rate below 60 beats per minute. Identification of the cardiac rhythm and any conduction disturbances is essential, and help with this can be found in Chapter 3.

Problems to consider in the bradycardic patient are:

- sinus bradycardia
- sick sinus syndrome
- second- and third-degree AV block
- 'escape' rhythms
  - AV junctional escape rhythm
  - ventricular escape rhythms
  - asystole.

Sinus bradycardia (p. 34) can be normal, for example in athletes during sleep, but in others may indicate an underlying problem. The differential diagnosis and treatment are discussed in Chapter 3.

Sick sinus syndrome (p. 38) is the coexistence of sinus bradycardia with episodes of sinus arrest and sinoatrial block. Patients may also have episodes of paroxysmal tachycardia, giving rise to the tachy-brady syndrome. This is discussed further on p. 39.

In **second-degree AV block** (p. 60) some atrial impulses fail to be conducted to the ventricles, and this can lead to bradycardia. In **third-degree AV block**, no atrial impulses can reach the ventricles; in response, the ventricles usually develop an 'escape' rhythm (see below). It is important to remember that AV block can coexist with *any* atrial rhythm.

Escape rhythms (p. 61) are a form of 'safety net' to maintain a heart beat if the normal mechanism of impulse generation fails or is blocked. They may also appear during episodes of severe sinus bradycardia. The distinction between AV junctional and ventricular escape rhythms is discussed in Chapter 3.

Asystole (p. 244) implies the absence of ventricular activity, and so the heart rate is zero. Asystole is a medical emergency and requires immediate diagnosis and treatment if the patient is to survive. A management algorithm can be found in Fig. 16.6.

As well as arrhythmias and conduction disturbances causing bradycardia, also consider the effects that certain **drugs** have on rhythms which usually cause normal or fast heart rates. For example, patients with atrial fibrillation (which, untreated, causes a *tachycardia*) can develop a ***bradycardia*** when commenced on antiarrhythmic drugs. Drugs that commonly slow the heart rate (**negatively chronotropic**) are listed in Table 2.1. A thorough review of all the patient's current and recent medications is therefore essential. The first step in managing a bradycardia is to assess the

Table 2.1 Negatively chronotropic drugs

- Beta blockers (do not forget eye drops)
- Some calcium antagonists, e.g. verapamil, diltiazem
- Digoxin
- Adenosine

DRUG POINT

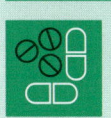

A complete drug history is essential in any patient with an abnormal ECG.

urgency of the situation. Ask the patient about symptoms (dizziness, syncope, falls, fatigue, breathlessness, chest pain and palpitations) and perform a thorough examination, looking particularly for evidence of haemodynamic disturbance (hypotension, cardiac failure and poor peripheral perfusion).

Use the history, examination and further investigations (e.g. plasma electrolytes, thyroid function tests) to identify any underlying cause and correct it where possible:

- Discontinue or reduce the dose of responsible drugs.
- Identify abnormal cardiac rhythms.
- Identify and treat hypothyroidism.

When bradycardia is severe and symptomatic, more urgent treatment is required:

- atropine, 300–600 μg given slowly intravenously (do not exceed 3 mg in 24 h).

A second-line agent is:

- isoprenaline, 0.5–10 μg/min by intravenous infusion.

However, insertion of a temporary pacemaker is preferable to prolonged infusions of isoprenaline, and so this drug should only be used as a short-term measure while arranging for temporary pacing.

Chronic bradycardia may be an indication for a permanent pacemaker, particularly when it is causing symptoms or haemodynamic disturbance. Referral to a cardiologist is recommended.

SEEK HELP

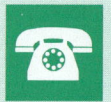

Bradycardias may require pacing, especially if symptomatic. Seek the advice of a cardiologist, without delay.

IS THE HEART RATE ABOVE 100 BEATS PER MINUTE?

Tachycardia is arbitrarily defined as a heart rate above 100 beats per minute. When a patient presents with a tachycardia, you must begin by identifying the cardiac rhythm. Consult Chapter 3 for specific descriptions of how to recognize and manage each rhythm.

You can begin the process of identification by checking whether the QRS complexes are:

- broad (> 3 small squares)
- narrow (< 3 small squares).

Narrow-complex tachycardias always arise from above the ventricles; that is, they are supraventricular in origin. The possibilities are:

- sinus tachycardia
- atrial tachycardia
- atrial flutter
- atrial fibrillation
- AV re-entry tachycardias.

All of these are discussed in detail in Chapter 3.

Broad QRS complexes can occur if normal electrical impulses are conducted abnormally or 'aberrantly' to the ventricles. This delays ventricular activation, widening the QRS complex. Any of the supraventricular tachycardias listed above can also present as a **broad-complex tachycardia** if aberrant conduction is present.

Broad-complex tachycardia should also make you think of ventricular arrhythmias:

- ventricular tachycardia
- accelerated idioventricular rhythm
- torsades de pointes.

Each of these is discussed in Chapter 3, and advice on how to distinguish between ventricular tachycardia (VT) and supraventricular tachycardia (SVT) can be found on p. 73.

Ventricular fibrillation (VF) is hard to categorize. The chaotic nature of the underlying ventricular activity can give rise to a variety of ECG appearances, but all have the characteristic of being unpredictable and chaotic. Ventricular fibrillation is a medical emergency and so it is important that you can recognize it immediately; you should study Chapter 16 if you are not confident in doing so.

The management of tachycardia depends upon the underlying rhythm, and the treatment of the different arrhythmias is detailed in Chapter 3. The first step, as with managing a bradycardia, is to assess the urgency of the situation.

Clues to the nature of the arrhythmia may be found in the patient's history. Ask the patient about how any palpitations start and stop (sudden or gradual), whether there are any situations in which they are more likely to happen (e.g. during exercise, lying quietly in bed), how long they last and whether there are any associated symptoms (dizziness, syncope, falls, fatigue, breathlessness and chest pain). Also ask the patient to 'tap out' how the palpitations feel – this will give you clues as to the rate (fast or slow) and rhythm (regular or irregular).

You must also enquire about symptoms of related disorders (e.g. hyperthyroidism) and obtain a list of current medications. Check for any drugs (e.g. salbutamol) that can increase the heart rate (**positively chronotropic**). Do not forget to ask about caffeine intake (coffee, tea and cola drinks).

A thorough examination is always important, looking for evidence of haemodynamic disturbance (hypotension, cardiac failure and poor peripheral perfusion) and coexistent disorders (e.g. a thyroid goitre).

Use the history, examination and further investigations (e.g. plasma electrolytes, thyroid function tests) to reach a diagnosis. A 24-h ambulatory ECG recording may be helpful if circumstances permit it.

In an emergency, every effort must be made to diagnose and correct the rhythm as quickly as possible. If the diagnosis is unclear and the patient needs immediate treatment, most tachycardias will respond to DC cardioversion. Do not hesitate to seek the urgent advice of a cardiologist if circumstances permit.

> ### ACT QUICKLY
> Tachycardia causing haemodynamic disturbance requires urgent diagnosis and treatment.

Summary

To assess the heart rate, ask the following questions:

1. Is the heart rate below 60 beats per minute?

If 'yes', consider:
- Sinus bradycardia
- Sick sinus syndrome
- Second- and third-degree AV block
- Escape rhythms
    - AV junctional escape rhythm
    - ventricular escape rhythms
- Asystole
- Drug-induced condition

2. Is the heart rate above 100 beats per minute?

If 'yes', consider:
- Narrow-complex tachycardia
    - sinus tachycardia
    - atrial tachycardia
    - atrial flutter
    - atrial fibrillation
    - AV re-entry tachycardias
- Broad-complex tachycardia
    - narrow-complex tachycardia with aberrant conduction
    - ventricular tachycardia
    - accelerated idioventricular rhythm
    - torsades de pointes

3

RHYTHM

To identify the cardiac rhythm with confidence you need to examine a rhythm strip – a prolonged recording of the ECG from just one lead, usually lead II (Fig. 3.1). Most modern ECG machines automatically include a rhythm strip at the bottom of a 12-lead ECG. If your machine does not, make sure you have recorded one yourself. The diagnosis of rhythm abnormalities may only become apparent when you examine 12 or more consecutive complexes.

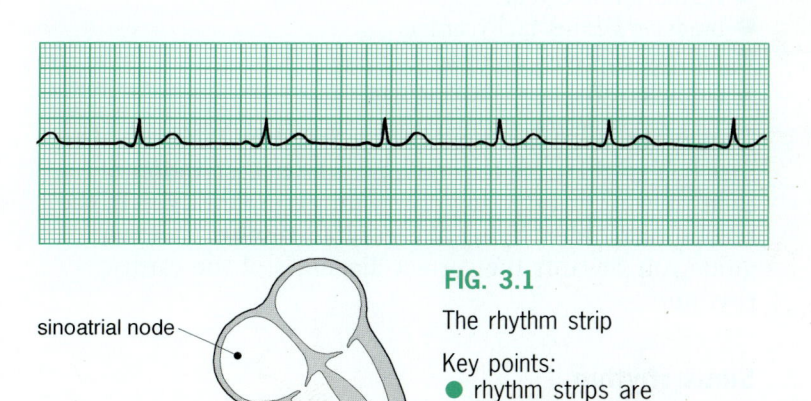

FIG. 3.1

The rhythm strip

Key points:
- rhythm strips are prolonged recordings from a single lead, often lead II
- this rhythm strip shows sinus rhythm

sinoatrial node

Even with a rhythm strip, however, the diagnosis of abnormal cardiac rhythms is not always easy, and some of the more complex arrhythmias can tax the skills of even the most experienced cardiologist. It is appropriate, therefore, to begin this chapter with the following warning:

SEEK HELP

If in doubt about a patient's cardiac rhythm, do not hesitate to seek the advice of a cardiologist.

This advice is particularly important if the patient is haemodynamically compromised by the arrhythmia, or if you are contemplating treatment of any kind.

There are many ways in which one can approach the identification of arrhythmias, and this is reflected in the numerous ways in which they can be categorized:

- regular vs irregular
- bradycardias vs tachycardias
- narrow complex vs broad complex
- supraventricular vs ventricular.

The common cardiac rhythms are listed in Table 3.1. The first half of this chapter contains a brief description of each rhythm in turn, together with example ECGs. In the second half, **'Identifying the cardiac rhythm'**, we will guide you towards the correct diagnosis of the cardiac rhythm.

Sinus rhythm

Sinus rhythm is the normal cardiac rhythm, in which the sinoatrial node acts as the natural pacemaker, discharging 60–100 times per minute (Fig. 3.2).

RHYTHM 33

Table 3.1 Cardiac rhythms

- SA nodal rhythms
  - sinus rhythm
  - sinus bradycardia
  - sinus tachycardia
  - sinus arrhythmia
  - sick sinus syndrome
- Atrial rhythms
  - atrial tachycardia
  - atrial flutter
  - atrial fibrillation
- AV junctional rhythms
- AV re-entry tachycardias
- Ventricular rhythms
  - ventricular tachycardia
  - accelerated idioventricular rhythm
  - torsades de pointes
  - ventricular fibrillation
- Conduction disturbances
- Escape rhythms
- Ectopic beats

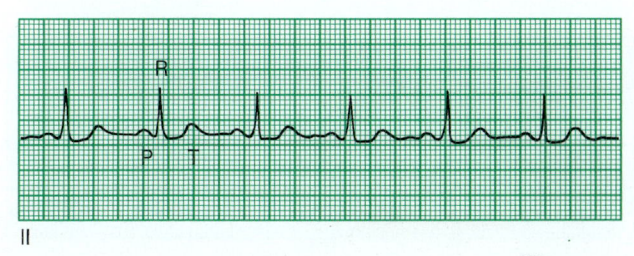

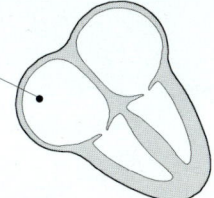

FIG. 3.2

Sinus rhythm

Key points:
- heart rate is 80 per minute
- P waves are upright (lead II)
- QRS complex after every P wave

34 MAKING SENSE OF THE ECG

The characteristic features of sinus rhythm are:

- Heart rate is 60–100 beats per minute.
- The P wave is upright in lead II and inverted in lead aVR.
- Every P wave is followed by a QRS complex.

If the patient is in sinus rhythm, move on to determine the cardiac axis (Chapter 4). If not, continue reading this chapter to diagnose the rhythm.

Sinus bradycardia

Sinus bradycardia is sinus rhythm with a heart rate of less than 60 beats per minute (Fig. 3.3).

The characteristic features of sinus bradycardia are:

- Heart rate is *less than* 60 beats per minute.
- The P wave is upright in lead II and inverted in lead aVR.
- Every P wave is followed by a QRS complex.

It is unusual for sinus bradycardia to be slower than 40 beats per minute – any slower and you should consider an

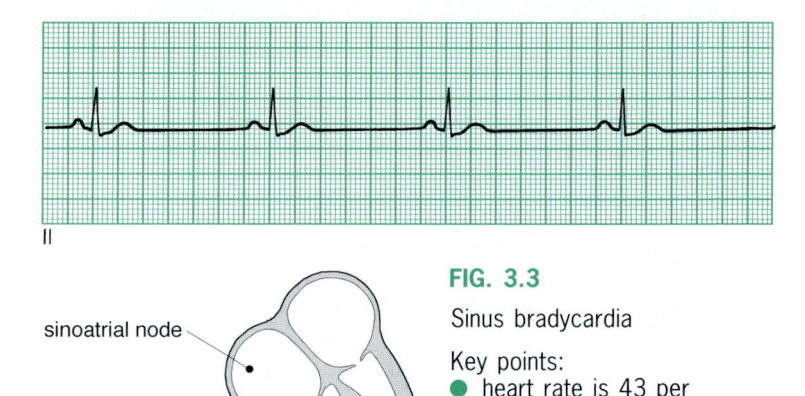

FIG. 3.3

Sinus bradycardia

Key points:
- heart rate is 43 per minute
- P waves are upright (lead II)
- QRS complex after every P wave

alternative cause, such as heart block (p. 60). Sinus bradycardia can be a normal finding, for example in athletes or during sleep. However, always consider the following possible causes:

- drugs (e.g. digoxin, beta blockers – including eye drops)
- ischaemic heart disease and myocardial infarction
- hypothyroidism
- hypothermia
- electrolyte abnormalities
- obstructive jaundice
- uraemia
- raised intracranial pressure
- sick sinus syndrome.

If the sinus bradycardia is severe, or if sinus arrest or sinoatrial block are prolonged, escape beats and escape rhythms may occur.

The management of bradycardia (of any cause) is discussed in detail on p. 24.

Sinus tachycardia

Sinus tachycardia is sinus rhythm with a heart rate of greater than 100 beats per minute (Fig. 3.4).

The characteristic features of sinus tachycardia are:

- Heart rate is *greater than* 100 beats per minute
- The P wave is upright in lead II and inverted in lead aVR.
- Every P wave is followed by a QRS complex.

It is rare for sinus tachycardia to exceed 180 beats per minute, except in fit athletes. At this heart rate, it may be difficult to differentiate the P waves from the T waves, so the rhythm can be mistaken for an atrioventricular nodal re-entry tachycardia.

Physiological causes of a sinus tachycardia include anything which stimulates the sympathetic nervous system – anxiety,

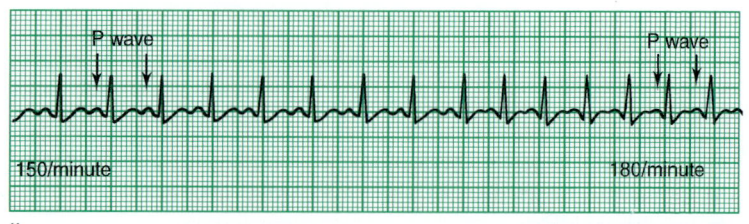

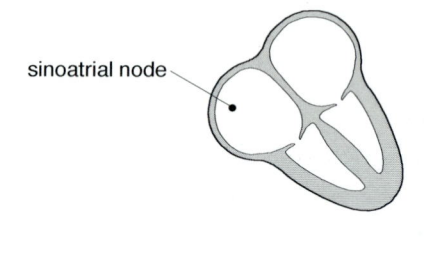

FIG. 3.4

Sinus tachycardia

Key points:
- heart rate is 150–180 per minute
- P waves are upright (lead II)
- QRS complex after every P wave

pain, fear, fever or exercise. Always consider the following causes too:

- drugs, e.g. adrenaline, atropine, salbutamol (do not forget inhalers and nebulizers), caffeine
- ischaemic heart disease and acute myocardial infarction
- heart failure
- pulmonary embolism
- fluid loss
- anaemia
- hyperthyroidism.

The management of sinus tachycardia is that of the cause. When a patient has an **appropriate** tachycardia (compensating for low blood pressure, such as in fluid loss or anaemia), slowing it with beta blockers can lead to disastrous decompensation. It is the underlying problem that needs addressing. However, if the sinus tachycardia is **inappropriate**, as in anxiety or hyperthyroidism, treatment with beta blockers may be helpful.

WARNING

In sinus tachycardia, never use a beta blocker to slow the heart rate until you have established the cause.

Sinus arrhythmia

Sinus arrhythmia is the variation in heart rate that is seen during inspiration and expiration (Fig. 3.5).

The characteristic features of sinus arrhythmia are:

- Every P wave is followed by a QRS complex.
- Heart rate varies with respiration.

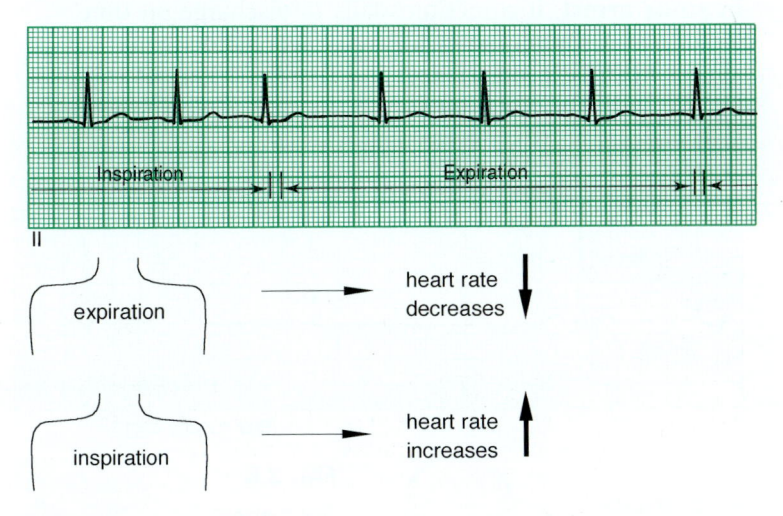

FIG. 3.5

Sinus arrhythmia

Key points:
- heart rate is 75 per minute during expiration
- heart rate is 90 per minute during inspiration

The heart rate normally increases during inspiration, as a reflex response to the increased volume of blood returning to the heart. Sinus arrhythmia is uncommon after the age of 40 years. The condition is harmless and no tests or treatment are necessary.

Sick sinus syndrome

As the name suggests, sick sinus syndrome is a collection of impulse generation and conduction problems related to dysfunction of the sinus node. Any, or all, of the following problems may be seen in a patient with the syndrome:

- sinus bradycardia
- sinus arrest
- sinoatrial block.

Sinus bradycardia has already been described (p. 34). The sinus node is normally a very reliable pacemaker. However, in **sinus arrest**, it sometimes fails to discharge on time – looking at a rhythm strip, a P wave will suddenly fail to appear in the expected place, and there is a gap, of variable length, until the sinus node fires and a P wave appears (Fig. 3.6).

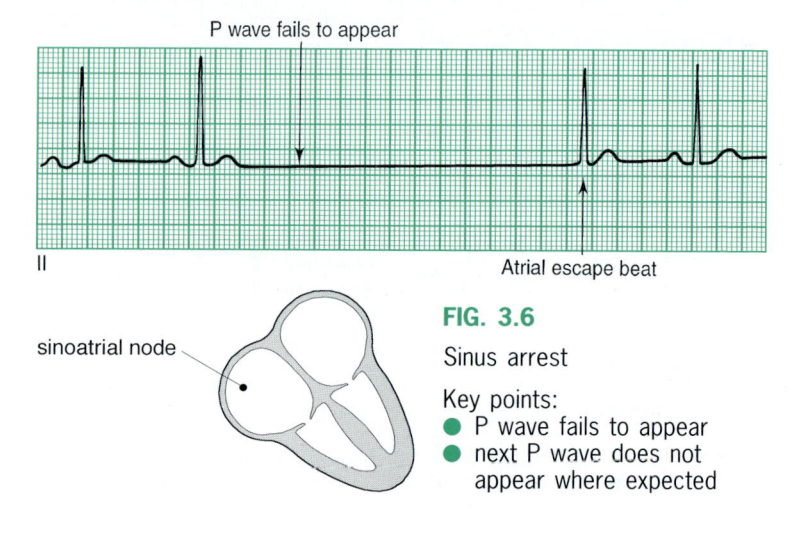

FIG. 3.6

Sinus arrest

Key points:
- P wave fails to appear
- next P wave does not appear where expected

FIG. 3.7

Sinoatrial block

Key points:
- P wave fails to appear
- next P wave appears where expected

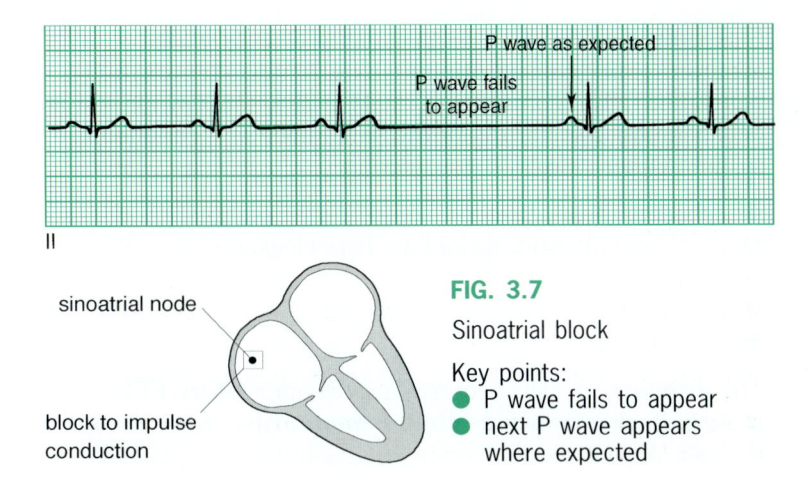

In **sinoatrial block**, the sinus node depolarizes as normal, but the impulse fails to reach the atria. A P wave fails to appear in the expected place, but the next one usually appears exactly where it is expected (Fig. 3.7).

If the sinus bradycardia is severe, or if sinus arrest or sinoatrial block are prolonged, escape beats and escape rhythms may occur. Sick sinus syndrome may also coexist with:

- certain paroxysmal tachycardias
  - atrial fibrillation (p. 44)
  - atrial flutter (p. 42)
  - atrial tachycardia (p. 40)
- AV nodal conduction disorders (p. 60).

The association of sick sinus syndrome with paroxysmal tachycardias is called **tachycardia–bradycardia** (or **'tachy-brady') syndrome**. The tachycardias often emerge as an escape rhythm in response to an episode of bradycardia. Evidence for abnormal AV nodal conduction often become apparent when a patient with tachy-brady syndrome develops atrial fibrillation with a slow ventricular response – the AV node fails to conduct the atrial impulses at the usual high rate.

Sick sinus syndrome, and the associated tachy-brady syndrome, may cause symptoms of dizziness, fainting and palpitations. The commonest cause of sick sinus syndrome is degeneration and fibrosis of the sinus node and conducting system. Other causes to consider are:

- ischaemic heart disease
- drugs (e.g. digoxin, quinidine, beta blockers)
- cardiomyopathy
- amyloidosis
- myocarditis.

The diagnosis usually requires a 24-h ambulatory ECG recording, also known as **Holter monitoring**. Asymptomatic patients do not require treatment. Symptomatic patients need consideration for a permanent pacemaker (Chapter 14). This is particularly important if they also have paroxysmal tachycardias that require antiarrhythmic drugs (which can worsen the episodes of bradycardia). Paroxysmal tachycardias which arise as escape rhythms in response to episodes of bradycardia may also improve as a consequence of pacing. Referral to a cardiologist is therefore recommended.

Atrial tachycardia

Atrial tachycardia differs from sinus tachycardia in that the impulses are generated by an ectopic focus somewhere within the atrial myocardium rather than the sinus node (Fig. 3.8).

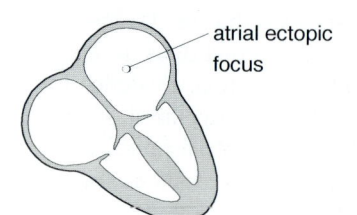

FIG. 3.8

Abnormal atrial focus

Key points:
- the abnormal focus means the spread of depolarization through the atria follows an abnormal route

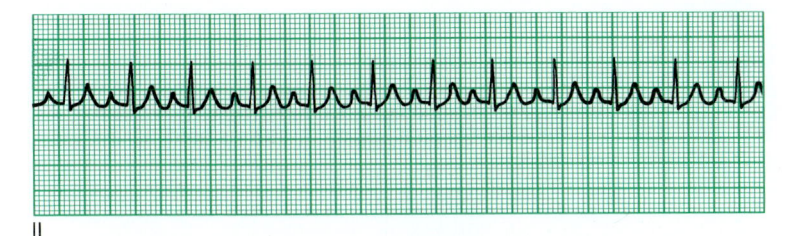

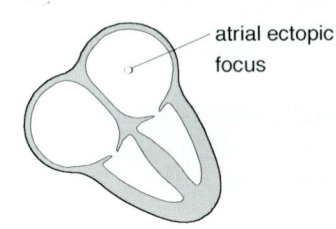

FIG. 3.9

Atrial tachycardia

Key points:
- heart rate is 125 per minute
- abnormally shaped P waves

This results in a rhythm strip with the following characteristic features (Fig. 3.9):

- heart rate greater than 100 beats per minute
- abnormally shaped P waves.

The atrial (P wave) rate is usually 120–250 per minute; above atrial rates of 200 per minute, the AV node struggles to keep up with impulse conduction and AV block may occur. The combination of atrial tachycardia with AV block is particularly common in digoxin toxicity. If the patient is not taking digoxin, then consider:

- ischaemic heart disease
- rheumatic heart disease
- cardiomyopathy
- sick sinus syndrome (p. 38).

For details on how to manage digoxin toxicity, see the section on digoxin in Chapter 9 (p. 174) If digoxin is not the cause, it can be used to control the ventricular response, as can verapamil or a beta blocker.

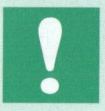

> **WARNING**
>
> **Never** give verapamil to a patient who is taking a beta blocker (or vice versa). A severe bradycardia can result.

Atrial flutter

Atrial flutter may share the same mechanism as atrial tachycardia (an ectopic atrial focus), or result from depolarization circling the right atrium (Fig. 3.10).

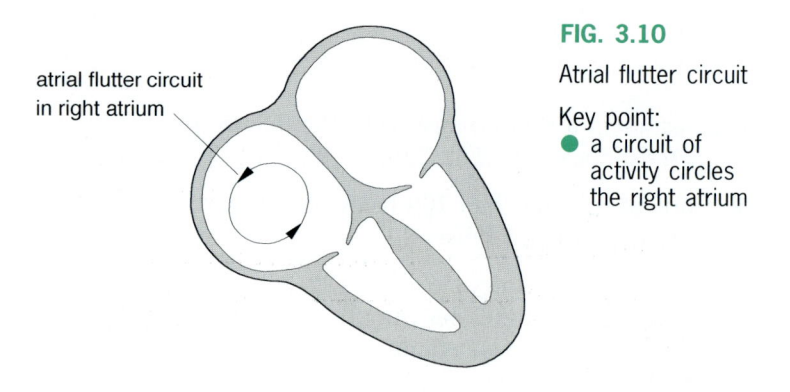

FIG. 3.10

Atrial flutter circuit

Key point:
- a circuit of activity circles the right atrium

Atrial flutter differs from atrial tachycardia in that the atrial (P wave) rate is higher, usually 250–350 per minute and often almost exactly 300 per minute. The AV node cannot keep up with such a high atrial rate and AV block occurs. This is most commonly 2:1 block, where only alternate atrial impulses get through the AV node to initiate a QRS complex, although 3:1, 4:1 or variable degrees of block are also seen (Fig. 3.11).

Thus, the ventricular rate is less than the atrial rate, and is often 150, 100 or 75 per minute. You should always suspect

RHYTHM 43

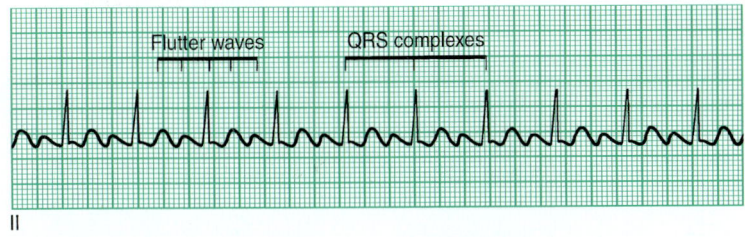

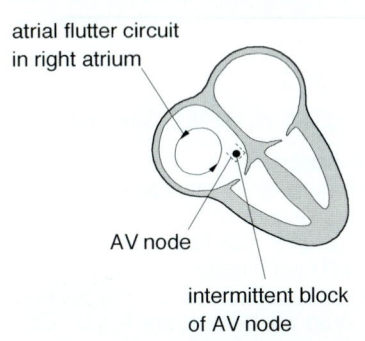

FIG. 3.11

Atrial flutter with 3:1 AV block

Key points:
- flutter waves at a rate of 300 per minute
- QRS complexes at a rate of 100 per minute
- therefore, 3:1 AV block is present

atrial flutter with 2:1 block when a patient has a regular tachycardia with a ventricular rate of around 150 per minute.

The rapid atrial rate gives a characteristic 'sawtooth' appearance to the baseline of the ECG. This can be made more apparent by carotid sinus massage. This will not terminate the atrial flutter, but will increase the degree of AV block, making the baseline easier to see by reducing the number of QRS complexes (Fig. 3.12).

Thus, the characteristic features of atrial flutter are:

- atrial rate around 300 per minute
- 'sawtooth' baseline
- AV block (usually 2:1, 3:1 or 4:1).

The causes of atrial flutter are the same as those of atrial fibrillation (see Table 3.2). Although digoxin, verapamil or beta blockers can be used simply to control the ventricular response, preferably you should aim to restore sinus rhythm. Drugs which can restore (and maintain) sinus rhythm include:

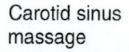

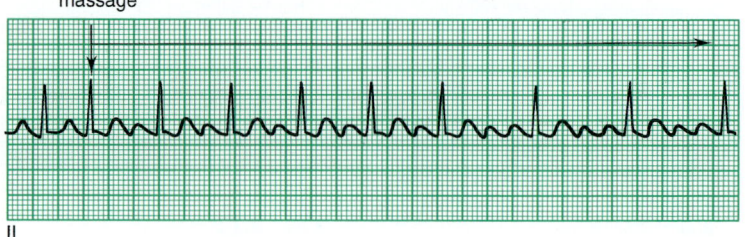

FIG. 3.12

The effect of carotid sinus massage

Key points:
- carotid sinus massage increases the degree of AV block
- the QRS rate falls from 150 to 110 per minute
- the flutter waves are more easily seen when there are fewer QRS complexes

- sotalol
- flecainide
- propafenone.

Atrial flutter can also be converted to sinus rhythm with DC cardioversion (p. 47) and overdrive atrial pacing (Chapter 14).

Atrial fibrillation

Atrial fibrillation is much commoner than atrial flutter, affecting 5–10% of elderly people. It may be permanent or, particularly in younger people, paroxysmal. The basis of atrial fibrillation is rapid, chaotic depolarization occurring throughout the atria. No P waves are seen and the ECG baseline consists of low-amplitude oscillations (fibrillation or 'f' waves). Although around 400–600 impulses reach the AV

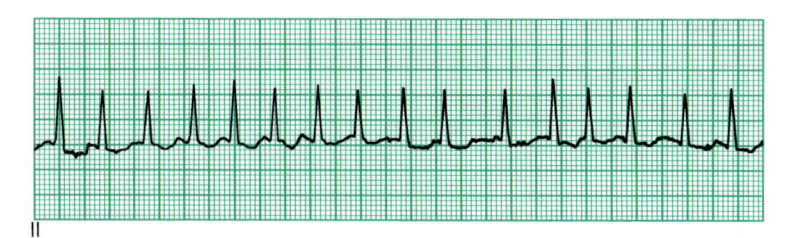

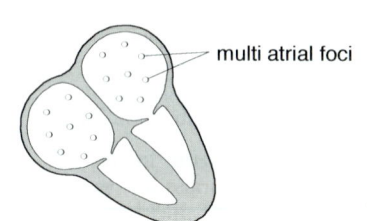

FIG. 3.13

Atrial fibrillation

Key points:
- irregularly irregular rhythm
- no P waves visible
- QRS rate is 170 per minute

node every minute, only 120–180 of these will reach the ventricles to produce QRS complexes. Transmission of the atrial impulses through the AV node is erratic, making the ventricular (QRS complex) rhythm 'irregularly irregular' (Fig. 3.13).

Thus, the characteristic features of atrial fibrillation are:

- absence of P waves
- irregularly irregular ventricular rhythm.

The erratic atrial depolarization leads to a failure of effective atrial contraction. Loss of the 'atrial kick' reduces ventricular filling and can lead to a fall of 10–15% in cardiac output.

Patients with atrial fibrillation will usually present with palpitations and/or symptoms of an underlying cause (Table 3.2). Systemic embolism is a significant risk in atrial fibrillation and may also be a presenting feature. Examination of the patient will reveal an irregularly irregular pulse.

Once atrial fibrillation has been diagnosed, a cause should be sought with a thorough patient history and examination. Thyroid function tests are essential as atrial fibrillation may

A permanent restoration of sinus rhythm can be difficult to achieve, particularly in patients who have been in atrial fibrillation for a long time. Certain drugs (sotalol, flecainide, propafenone and quinidine) can restore sinus rhythm, as can DC cardioversion (see box). Maintenance of sinus rhythm can be achieved with any of these drugs, but there is only around a 50:50 chance of sustaining sinus rhythm beyond 1 year. Amiodarone is probably more effective, but can lead to troublesome side-effects.

In paroxysmal atrial fibrillation, the aim should be to reduce embolization risk (as above) and reduce the likelihood of recurrent paroxysms. Sotalol, flecainide, propafenone and disopyramide may each be useful. Digoxin should be avoided as it does not help in paroxysmal atrial fibrillation, and may even make it worse.

Patients whose atrial fibrillation is resistant to treatment should be referred to a cardiologist.

Resistant atrial fibrillation

The non-pharmacological treatment of resistant atrial fibrillation includes:
- AV nodal ablation (to prevent conduction from the atria to the ventricles) with insertion of a permanent ventricular pacemaker;
- experimental surgical techniques to the atrial myocardium to redirect the flow of atrial impulses.

AV re-entry tachycardias

AV re-entry tachycardias can arise when there is a second connection between the atria and ventricles, in addition to the normal route of conduction via the AV node. The presence of two different routes creates the possibility that impulses can travel down one (anterograde conduction) and then back up the other (retrograde conduction). In doing so, an impulse can enter into a repeated cycle of activity, circling round the two pathways so that it repeatedly re-enters and activates the atria and ventricles in rapid succession (Fig. 3.14).

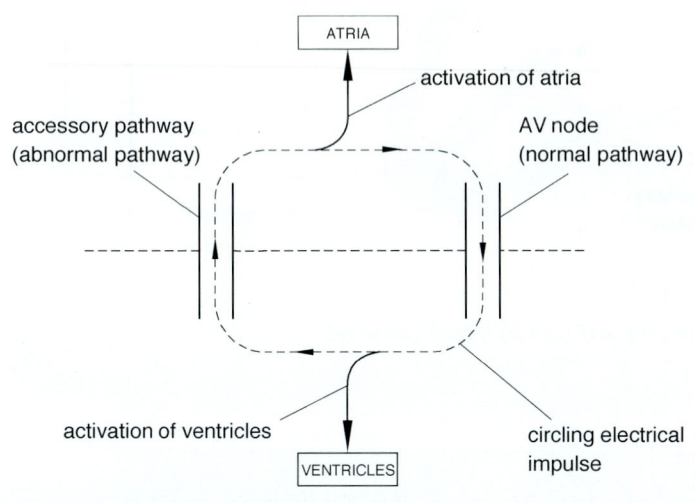

FIG. 3.14

Conduction around an AV re-entry circuit

The extra connection between atria and ventricles can be either an **accessory pathway**, anatomically separate from the AV node, or a **dual AV nodal pathway**, in which both pathways lie within the AV node but are electrically distinct (Fig. 3.15).

Accessory pathways are found in the Wolff–Parkinson–White (WPW) syndrome, described in Chapter 6, and patients are susceptible to episodes of **AV re-entry tachycardia**, with anterograde conduction via the AV node and retrograde conduction via the accessory pathway. During the tachycardia the delta wave is lost (Fig. 3.16). A re-entrant tachycardia taking the opposite route (down the accessory

50 MAKING SENSE OF THE ECG

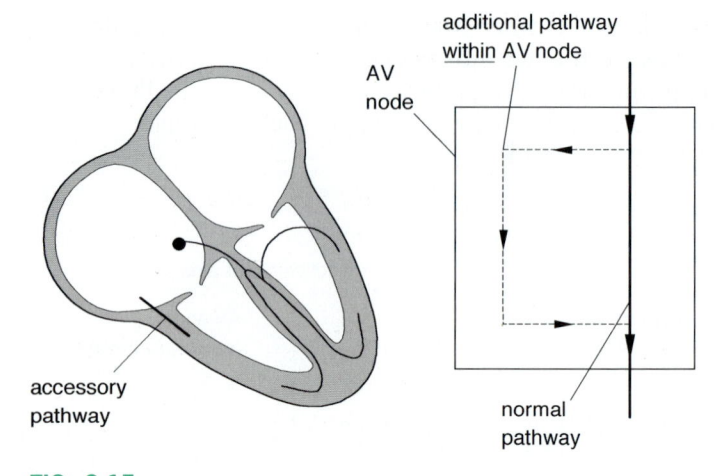

FIG. 3.15

Accessory and dual AV nodal pathways

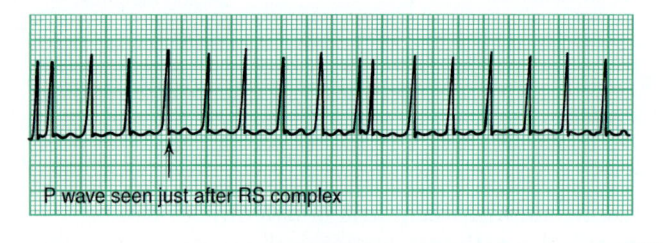

FIG. 3.16

AV re-entry tachycardia in WPW syndrome

Key points:
- ventricular rate is 188 per minute
- narrow RS complexes

pathway and up the AV node) is very rare, but when it does occur, only delta waves are seen (as the whole of the ventricular muscle is activated via the accessory pathway).

Patients with a dual AV nodal pathway are at risk of **AV nodal re-entry tachycardia**, in which anterograde conduction usually occurs down the normal AV nodal pathway and returns retrogradely via the abnormal additional pathway (Fig. 3.17).

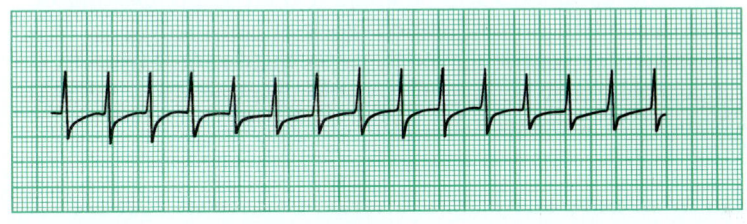

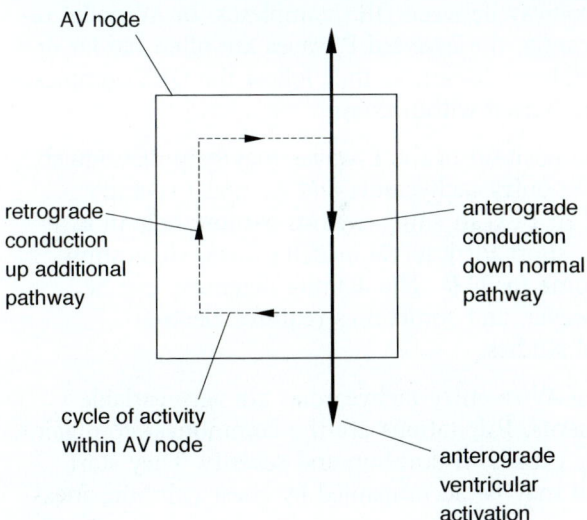

FIG. 3.17

AV nodal re-entry tachycardia

Key points:
- ventricular rate is 180 per minute
- narrow RS complexes

Both AV re-entry tachycardia and AV nodal re-entry tachycardia have the following characteristics:

- Heart rate is 130–250 beats per minute.
- There is one P wave per QRS complex (although P waves are not always clearly seen).
- There are regular QRS complexes.
- QRS complexes are narrow (in the absence of aberrant conduction).

The QRS complexes will be broad if there is pre-existing or rate-dependent bundle branch block. It can then be mistaken for ventricular tachycardia (p. 55). An earlier ECG, if available, may be helpful in determining whether a bundle branch block existed before the tachycardia (Fig. 3.18).

In AV re-entry tachycardia, inverted P waves (p. 102) are often seen halfway between QRS complexes. In AV nodal re-entry tachycardia, the inverted P waves are often harder or even impossible to discern as they follow the QRS complexes closely or are buried within them.

Although the position of the P waves may help distinguish between AV re-entry tachycardia and AV nodal re-entry tachycardia, an ECG in sinus rhythm is more helpful as it may reveal a short PR interval or delta wave, suggesting WPW syndrome (p. 111). The definite diagnosis can be difficult, however, and sometimes requires electrophysiological studies.

Symptoms of AV re-entry tachycardias are very variable between patients. Palpitations are the commonest complaint, and can vary greatly in duration and severity. They start suddenly and may be accompanied by chest pain, dizziness or syncope.

AV re-entry tachycardias can be terminated by blocking the AV node, thereby breaking the cycle of electrical activity. The **Valsalva manoeuvre** increases vagal inhibition of AV nodal conduction, thus slowing the AV nodal conduction and often

RHYTHM 53

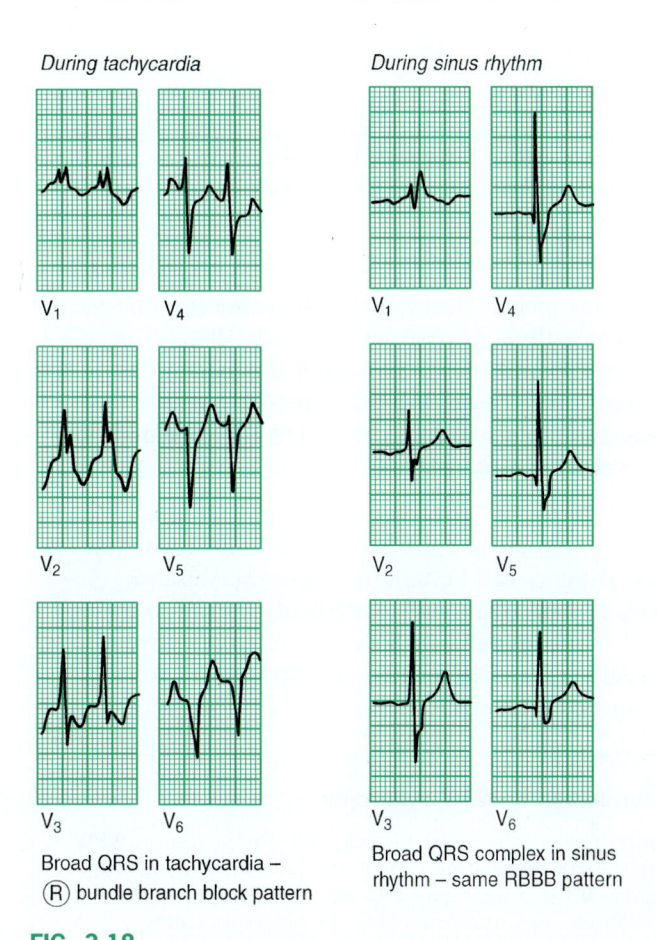

During tachycardia   *During sinus rhythm*

V₁   V₄   V₁   V₄

V₂   V₅   V₂   V₅

V₃   V₆   V₃   V₆

Broad QRS in tachycardia – Ⓡ bundle branch block pattern

Broad QRS complex in sinus rhythm – same RBBB pattern

FIG. 3.18

An earlier ECG can help diagnose pre-existing bundle branch block

terminating the tachycardia. Alternatively, you can perform **carotid sinus massage** (while monitoring the ECG) with the same aim. The technique of carotid sinus massage is illustrated in Fig. 3.12.

> **Valsalva manoeuvre**
>
> The Valsalva manoeuvre describes the action of forced expiration against a closed glottis. To perform it, patients should be asked to breathe in and then to strain for a few seconds with their breath held.

Drug treatments include intravenous **adenosine** (do not use if the patient has asthma or obstructive airways disease) or intravenous **verapamil** (not to be used if the patient has recently taken a beta blocker). If the patient is haemodynamically compromised, consider urgent **DC cardioversion** (p. 47) or **overdrive atrial pacing** (Chapter 14).

In the longer term, the arrhythmia does not require prophylactic treatment if episodes are brief and cause few symptoms. Patients can be taught to use the Valsalva manoeuvre. If drug treatment is required, referral to a cardiologist is recommended. Sotalol is often effective as a first-line agent but radiofrequency ablation via a cardiac catheter can be curative.

> **Atrial fibrillation in WPW syndrome**
>
> AV re-entry tachycardia is not the only arrhythmia seen in WPW syndrome. **Atrial fibrillation** can be precipitated by the re-entry tachycardia. If the patient goes into atrial fibrillation, conduction to the ventricles can occur via either the accessory pathway (which is commonest) or the AV node, or both. Conduction via the accessory pathway can cause a rapid and potentially lethal ventricular rate in response. Drugs that block the AV node (e.g. digoxin, verapamil or adenosine) are therefore **hazardous** in these patients as they will *increase* conduction down the accessory pathway. DC cardioversion is the treatment of choice if the patient is haemodynamically compromised. Recurrent episodes can be treated with drugs that slow conduction in the accessory pathway, such as sotalol, flecainide, disopyramide or amiodarone. Patients resistant to drug therapy should be considered for accessory pathway ablation.

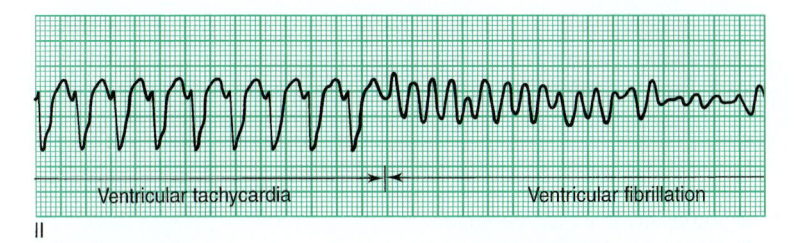

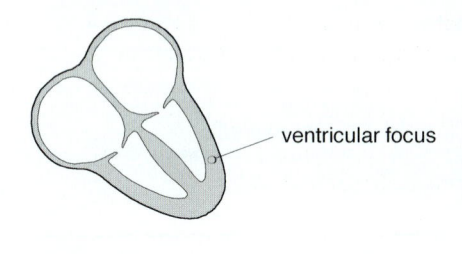

FIG. 3.19

Ventricular tachycardia (VT) and ventricular fibrillation (VF)

Key points:
- broad-complex tachycardia at a rate of 190 per minute (VT)
- degenerates into chaotic rhythm (VF)

Ventricular tachycardia

Ventricular tachycardia (VT) is a **broad-complex tachycardia**, defined as three or more successive ventricular beats at a heart rate above 120 beats per minute. Episodes can be self-terminating or can be sustained, or can degenerate into ventricular fibrillation (Fig. 3.19).

Characteristic features of VT are:

- ventricular rate above 120 per minute
- broad QRS complexes.

Sustained VT normally occurs at a heart rate of 150–250 per minute, but the diagnosis can be difficult. VT can be remarkably well tolerated and may not cause haemodynamic disturbance. Do *not* assume, therefore, that if the patient appears well then it is not VT. Help with distinguishing VT from arrhythmias with similar ECG appearances is given in the second half of this chapter.

The symptoms of ventricular tachycardia can vary from mild palpitations to dizziness, syncope and cardiac arrest. Always look for an underlying treatable cause (Table 3.3).

Table 3.3 Causes of ventricular tachycardia

- Acute myocardial infarction
- Ischaemic heart disease
- Hypertrophic cardiomyopathy
- Dilated cardiomyopathy
- Mitral valve prolapse
- Myocarditis
- Congenital heart disease (repaired or unrepaired)
- Electrolyte disturbance
- Proarrhythmic drugs
- Idiopathic

An episode of VT can be terminated using:

- drugs
- DC cardioversion
- pacing.

Choose the treatment according to the clinical state of the patient. When haemodynamic impairment is present, ventricular tachycardia becomes a medical emergency and warrants urgent DC cardioversion (p. 246).

ACT QUICKLY

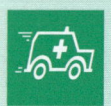

VT causing haemodynamic compromise is an emergency. Immediate diagnosis and treatment are required.

Stable patients can be cardioverted medically. Lignocaine is often the first-line agent, but alternatives include flecainide, sotalol, disopyramide and amiodarone. Overdrive right ventricular pacing (Chapter 14) is also effective but may precipitate ventricular fibrillation.

Long-term prophylaxis should be discussed with a cardiologist. It should be avoided for VT that occurred early in acute myocardial infarction. Effective drug treatments include sotalol (particularly when VT is exercise-related) and amiodarone. VT related to bradycardia should be treated by pacing. Ablation or surgery can be used to remove a ventricular focus identified by electrophysiological testing. Finally, automatic implantable cardiovertor defibrillator (AICD) devices can be implanted to deliver low energy DC shocks for recurrent episodes of VT (and VF).

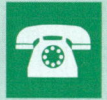

> **SEEK HELP**
>
> The management options for recurrent VT should be discussed with a cardiologist.

Accelerated idioventricular rhythm

Accelerated idioventricular rhythm is a slow form of ventricular tachycardia, with a heart rate of less than 120 beats per minute (Fig. 3.20).

It is usually seen in the setting of an acute myocardial infarction and is benign. No treatment is necessary.

Torsades de pointes

Torsades de pointes is an unusual variant of VT that is associated with a long QT interval (p. 200). Its name derives from the characteristic undulating pattern on the ECG, with a variation in the direction of the QRS axis (Fig. 3.21).

It can occur with certain antiarrhythmic drug treatments, electrolyte abnormalities and hereditary syndromes (see

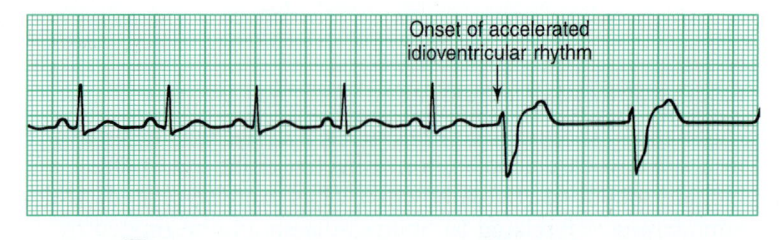

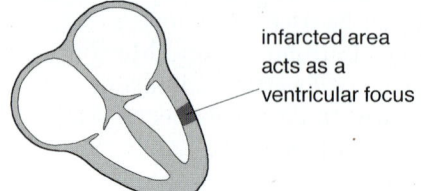

FIG. 3.20

Accelerated idioventricular rhythm

Key points:
- broad QRS complexes
- heart rate is 60 per minute

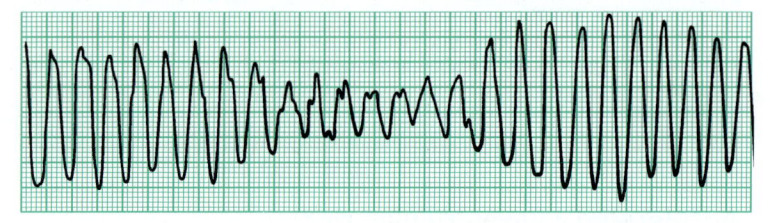

FIG. 3.21

Torsades de pointes

Key points:
- broad-complex tachycardia (rate is 270 per minute)
- variation in QRS axis

Chapter 11). As it carries a risk of precipitating ventricular fibrillation, urgent assessment is warranted, with referral to a cardiologist if necessary. Any causative drugs need to be identified and withdrawn, and electrolyte abnormalities corrected.

In an emergency, torsades de pointes can be treated with beta blockers, magnesium and temporary pacing which increases the heart rate and thereby shortens the QT interval. In the congenital long QT syndromes, beta blockers or left cervical sympathectomy are indicated to interrupt the sympathetic supply to the heart.

> **SEEK HELP**
>
> Torsades de pointes can cause ventricular fibrillation. Urgent referral to a cardiologist is recommended.

Ventricular fibrillation

Untreated ventricular fibrillation is a rapidly fatal arrhythmia. It therefore requires immediate diagnosis and treatment. Turn to p. 247 of Chapter 16 to find the emergency management algorithm for this arrhythmia.

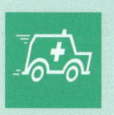

> **ACT QUICKLY**
>
> Ventricular fibrillation is a medical emergency. Immediate diagnosis and treatment are essential.

VF is most commonly seen in the setting of an acute myocardial infarction. Always check for electrolyte or acid–base abnormalities following an episode of VF. A single episode of **primary VF** (occurring within 48 h of an infarction), once corrected by DC shock, does not require prophylactic treatment.

Recurrent episodes of VF, or **secondary VF** (after 48 h), merit prophylaxis with lignocaine. Long-term prophylaxis is the same as for VT (see p. 57).

Conduction disturbances

The normal conduction of impulses from the SA node to the ventricles was described in Chapter 1. Block can occur at many different points along this route (Fig. 3.22).

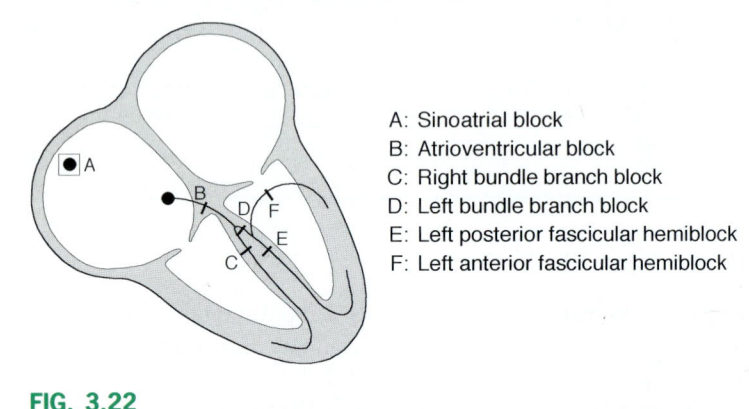

A: Sinoatrial block
B: Atrioventricular block
C: Right bundle branch block
D: Left bundle branch block
E: Left posterior fascicular hemiblock
F: Left anterior fascicular hemiblock

FIG. 3.22
Regions where conduction blocks can occur

In **sinoatrial (SA) block**, the SA node depolarizes as normal, but the impulse fails to reach the atria. A P wave fails to appear in the expected place, but the next one usually appears exactly on time. An example is shown in Fig. 3.7.

Atrioventricular (AV) block (Chapter 6) is of three degrees of severity. First-degree AV block simply lengthens the PR interval by delaying conduction through the AV node. In second-degree AV block, some atrial impulses fail to be conducted to the ventricles. In third-degree AV block, there is no conduction between atria and ventricles.

Further down the conducting system, **bundle branch block** can affect either the left or right bundle branch. Sometimes only one of the two fascicles of the left bundle branch is affected. Any permutation of these is possible, and block of both bundle branches together is equivalent to third-degree

AV block, as no impulses will reach the ventricular myocardium. Bundle branch block is discussed on p. 144, and fascicular block on pp. 89 and 95.

Conduction disturbances are not always a consistent feature of the ECG. They can be rate-dependent, only appearing at high heart rates when compromised regions of the conducting system fail to keep pace with the conduction of impulses. The development of bundle branch block during a supraventricular tachycardia, for example, can give it the appearance of ventricular tachycardia (p. 73).

Conduction disturbances are important to recognize, not only because of their effects on the appearance of the ECG but also because escape rhythms can appear when there is complete block of normal conduction.

Escape rhythms

Escape rhythms are a form of 'safety net' for the heart. Without escape rhythms, complete failure of impulse generation or conduction at any time would lead to ventricular asystole and death. Instead, the heart has a number of subsidiary pacemakers that can take over if normal impulse generation or conduction fails.

The subsidiary pacemakers are located in the AV junction and the ventricular myocardium. If the AV junction fails to receive impulses, as a result of SA arrest or block (p. 38), or even during severe sinus bradycardia, it will take over as the cardiac pacemaker. The QRS complex(es) generated will have the same morphology as normal but at a slower rate of around 40–60 beats per minute (Fig. 3.23).

The AV junctional pacemaker will continue until it again starts to be inhibited by impulses from the SA node. If the AV junctional pacemaker fails, or its impulses are blocked, a ventricular pacemaker will take over. Its rhythm is even slower, at 15–40 beats per minute, and the QRS complexes will be broad (Fig. 3.24).

FIG. 3.23

AV junctional escape rhythm

Key points:
- heart rate is 43 per minute
- absent P waves
- narrow QRS complexes

AV junctional pacemaker

FIG. 3.24

Ventricular escape rhythm

Key points:
- heart rate is 33 per minute
- absent P waves
- broad QRS complexes

ventricular escape pacemaker

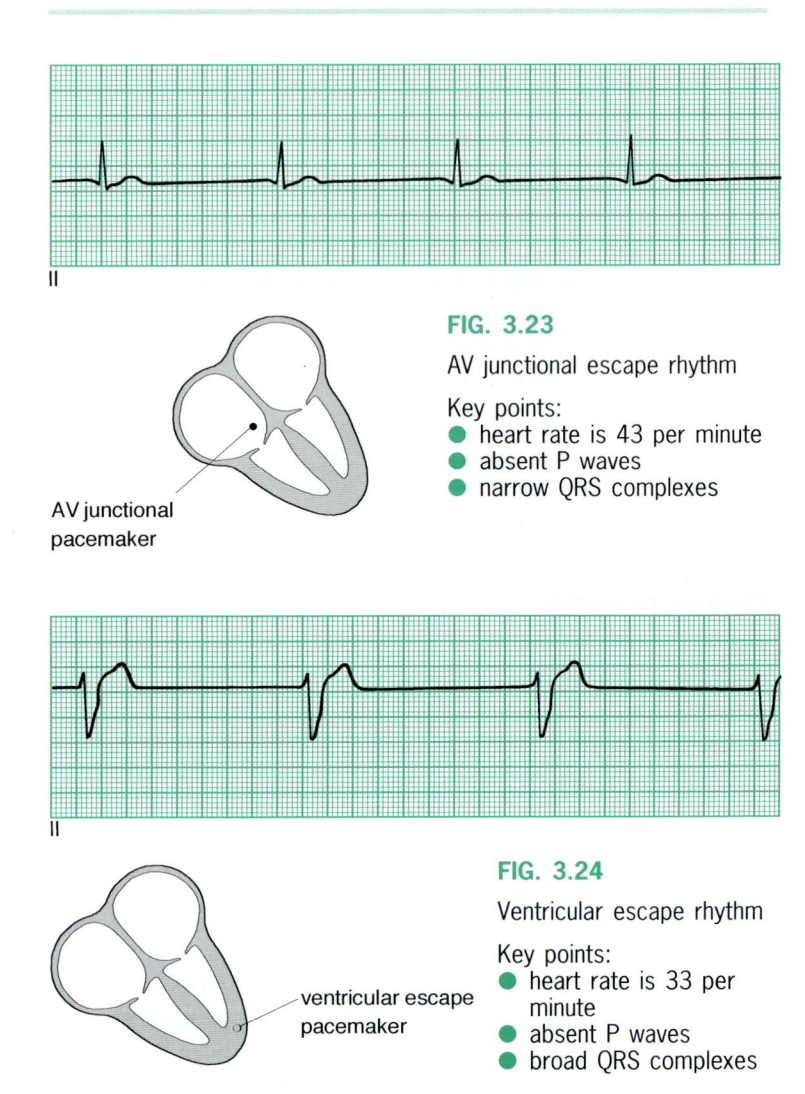

Because escape rhythms exist as a safety net, they must *not* be suppressed. Instead, you must identify why the escape rhythm has arisen (i.e. why normal impulse generation has failed or been blocked) and correct that underlying problem.

This will usually require a pacemaker, and should be discussed with a cardiologist.

Ectopic beats

In contrast to the QRS complexes of escape rhythms, which appear *later* than expected, ectopic beats appear *earlier* than expected. They can arise from any region of the heart, but are normally classified into atrial, AV junctional and ventricular ectopics. Ectopic beats are also called **extrasystoles** and **premature beats**.

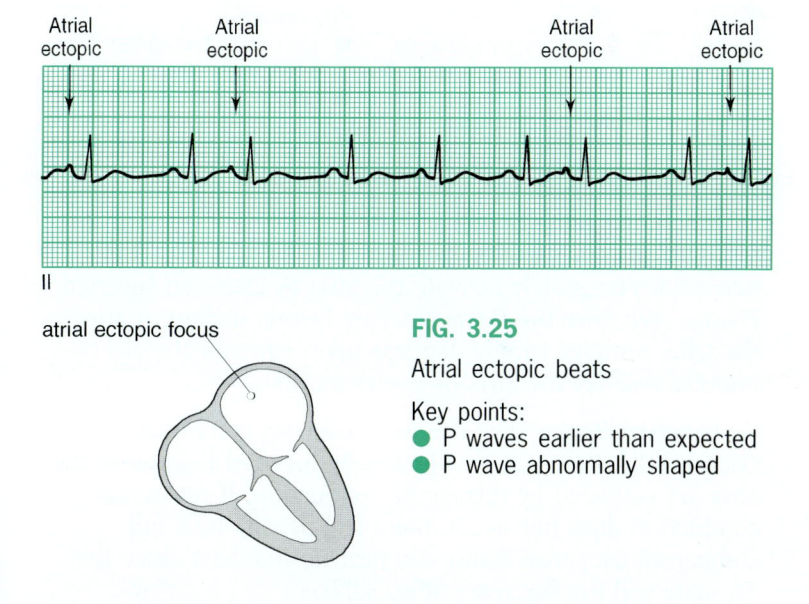

FIG. 3.25

Atrial ectopic beats

Key points:
- P waves earlier than expected
- P wave abnormally shaped

Atrial ectopics are identified by a P wave which appears earlier than expected and has an abnormal shape (Fig. 3.25). Although atrial ectopic beats will usually be conducted to the ventricles and give rise to a QRS complex, occasionally they may encounter a refractory AV node and fail to be conducted.

FIG. 3.26

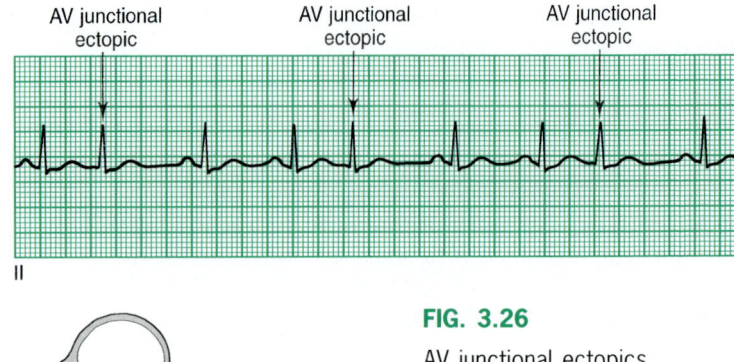

AV junctional ectopics

Key points:
- QRS complex earlier than expected
- QRS complex is narrow

AV junctional ectopics will activate the ventricles, giving rise to a QRS complex earlier than expected (Fig. 3.26). They may also retrogradely activate the atria to cause an inverted P wave. Whether the P wave occurs before, during or after the QRS complex simply depends upon whether the electrical impulse reaches the atria or ventricles first.

Ventricular ectopics give rise to broad QRS complexes. Occasionally, they will be followed by inverted P waves if the atria are activated by retrograde conduction. If retrograde conduction does not occur, there will usually be a full compensatory pause before the next normal beat since the SA node will not be 'reset' (Fig. 3.27).

Ventricular ectopics can occur at the same time as the T wave of the preceding beat. In the setting of an acute myocardial infarction, such 'R on T' ectopics can trigger ventricular arrhythmias.

Ventricular ectopics can be frequent. When one ectopic follows every normal beat, the term 'bigeminy' is used (Fig. 3.28).

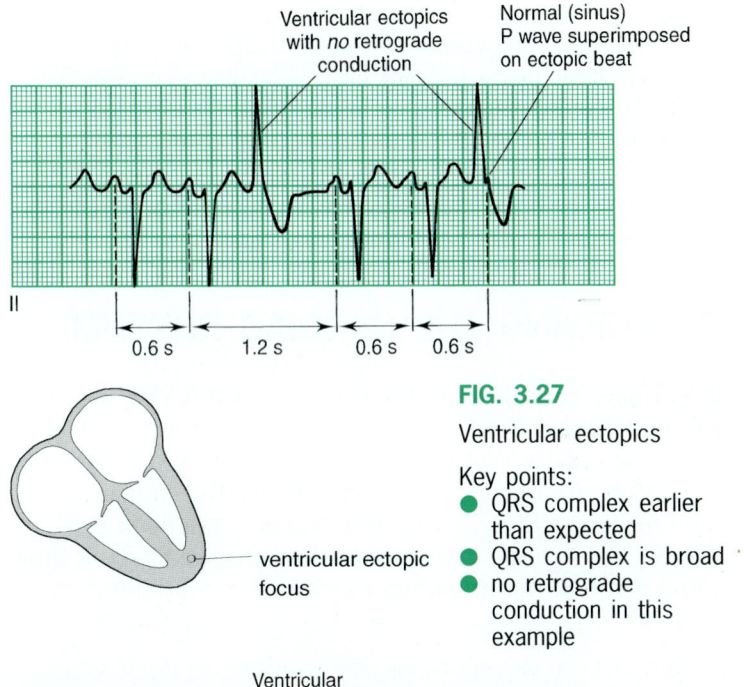

RHYTHM 65

Ventricular ectopics with *no* retrograde conduction

Normal (sinus) P wave superimposed on ectopic beat

II

0.6 s 1.2 s 0.6 s 0.6 s

FIG. 3.27

Ventricular ectopics

Key points:
- QRS complex earlier than expected
- QRS complex is broad
- no retrograde conduction in this example

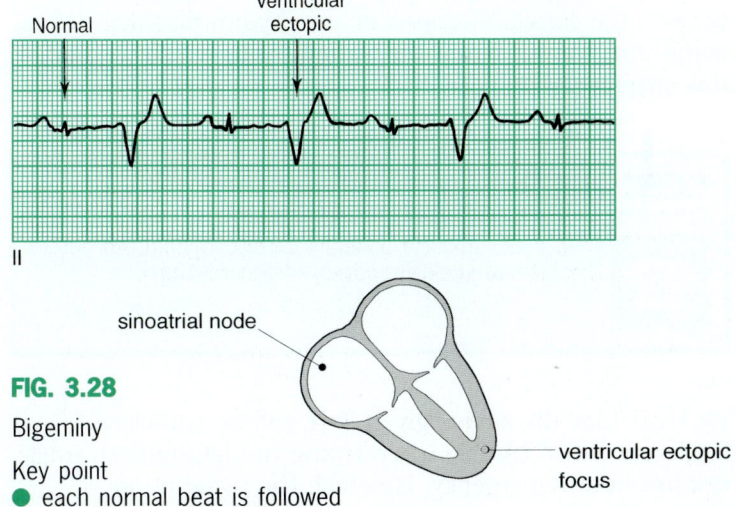

ventricular ectopic focus

Normal

Ventricular ectopic

II

sinoatrial node

FIG. 3.28

Bigeminy

Key point
- each normal beat is followed by a ventricular ectopic

ventricular ectopic focus

Despite the fact that some ventricular ectopics can precipitate fatal arrhythmias, routine treatment with antiarrhythmic drugs has not been shown to decrease mortality. Some patients may be significantly troubled by symptoms caused by the ectopic beat, the compensatory pause or the following sinus beat (usually a feeling of 'extra beats', 'missed beats' or 'heavy beats') and will benefit from using an antiarrhythmic agent.

IDENTIFYING THE CARDIAC RHYTHM

If you have read through the first part of this chapter, you will now have a good idea of the range of normal and abnormal cardiac rhythms, and their causes and treatment, and will be in a good position to identify the cardiac rhythm in any ECG. If you have turned straight to this section, we strongly recommend that you spend some time going through the preceding pages before continuing any further.

In this section, we will teach you a routine to guide you towards the correct diagnosis of any rhythm disorder. Before doing this, we will repeat the warning with which we started this chapter.

SEEK HELP

If in doubt about a patient's cardiac rhythm, do not hesitate to seek the advice of a cardiologist

We trust that the advice given here will be sufficient to keep you out of trouble when trying to identify the cardiac rhythm in an emergency. However, the recognition of some arrhythmias can be difficult, even for the specialist, and, if you are at all uncertain about the diagnosis, it is important that you seek expert help at the earliest opportunity.

When you analyse the cardiac rhythm, always keep in mind the two questions that you are trying to answer:

- Where does the impulse arise from?
  - sinoatrial (SA) node
  - atria
  - atrioventricular (AV) junction
  - ventricles.
- How is the impulse conducted?
  - normal conduction
  - accelerated conduction (e.g. WPW syndrome)
  - blocked conduction.

We will help you to narrow down the possible diagnoses with the following questions:

- Is the rhythm ventricular or supraventricular?
- Are P waves present?
- Is the rhythm regular or irregular?
- Is the rhythm a bradycardia or tachycardia?
- How do I distinguish between VT and SVT?

Is the rhythm ventricular or supraventricular?

By answering this question, you will already have narrowed down the origin of the impulse to one half of the heart. Ventricular rhythms are generated within the ventricular myocardium; supraventricular rhythms are generated anywhere up to (and including) the AV junction (Fig. 3.29).

Ventricular rhythms include the following:

- ventricular fibrillation
- ventricular tachycardia
- ventricular escape rhythms
- ventricular ectopics.

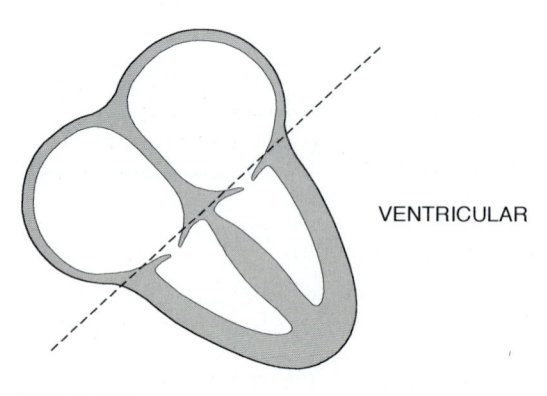

FIG. 3.29

Supraventricular vs ventricular rhythm

Key point:
- supraventricular applies to any structure above the ventricles (and electrically distinct from them)

You must be able to diagnose ventricular fibrillation at first sight, as it is rapidly fatal without immediate action. All the other ventricular rhythms have one property in common: they all produce **broad QRS complexes** (> 3 small squares).

However, supraventricular rhythms also produce broad QRS complexes if there is aberrant conduction (bundle branch block or an accessory pathway). When conduction is normal, supraventricular rhythms produce narrow QRS complexes. This is summarized in Table 3.4.

Table 3.4 Broad-complex vs narrow-complex rhythms

	Broad complex	Narrow complex
Supraventricular rhythm with normal conduction	✗	✓
Supraventricular rhythm with aberrant conduction	✓	✗
Ventricular rhythm	✓	✗

The distinction of VT and SVT is discussed specifically on p. 73.

Are P waves present?

The presence of P waves indicates atrial activity. By examining the P waves carefully, you can gain clues about the origin of atrial depolarization and how this relates to the ventricular (QRS complex) activity.

The shape of the P wave may provide a clue as to the origin of atrial depolarization (Chapter 5). Upright P waves in lead II suggest that depolarization originated in or near the SA node. Inverted P waves suggest an origin closer to, or within, the AV node (Fig. 3.30).

If every QRS complex is associated with a P wave, this indicates that the atria and ventricles are being activated by a common source. This is usually, but not necessarily, the SA node; AV junctional rhythms, for example, will also depolarize both atria and ventricles.

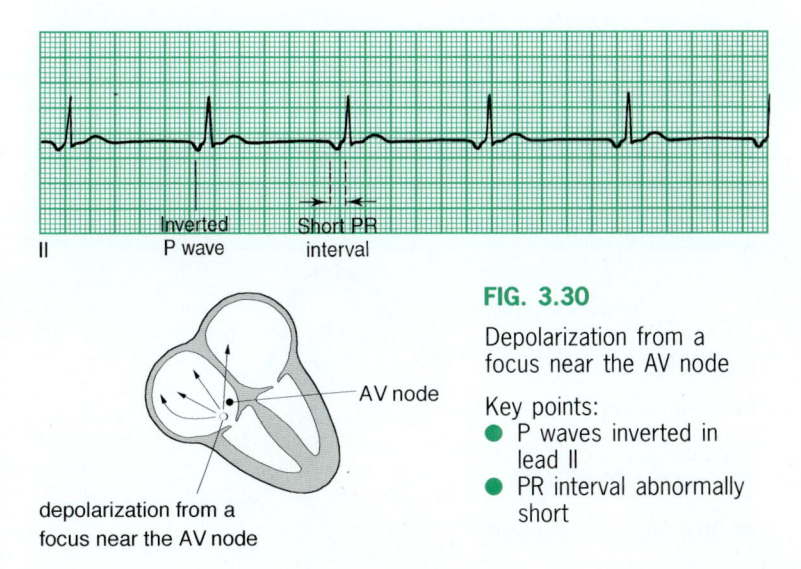

FIG. 3.30

Depolarization from a focus near the AV node

Key points:
- P waves inverted in lead II
- PR interval abnormally short

70 MAKING SENSE OF THE ECG

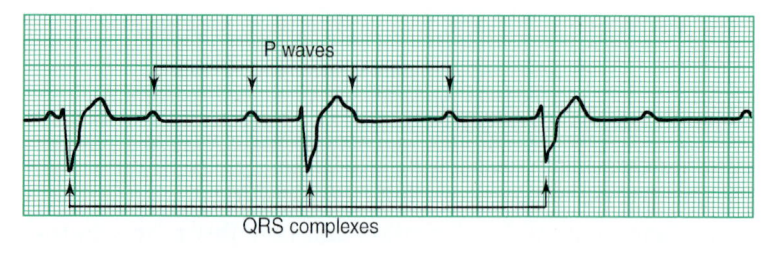

FIG. 3.31

Complete ('third-degree') AV block

Key points:
- P wave rate is 75 per minute
- QRS rate is 33 per minute

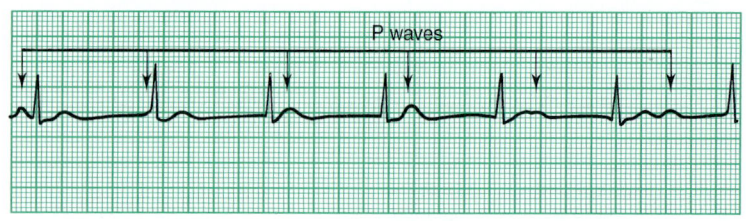

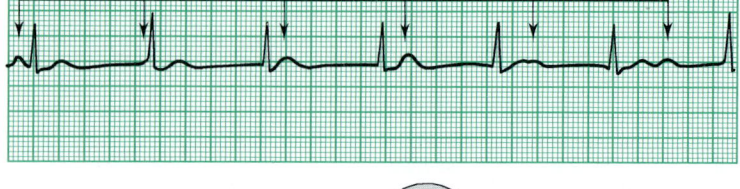

FIG. 3.32

AV dissociation

Key points:
- P wave rate 58 per minute
- QRS rate 65 per minute

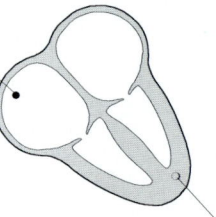

If there are more P waves than QRS complexes, conduction between atria and ventricles is being either *partly* blocked (with only some impulses getting through), or *completely* blocked (with the ventricles having developed their own escape rhythm). An example is shown in Fig. 3.31.

More QRS complexes than P waves indicate AV dissociation (p. 122), with the ventricles operating independently of the atria and at a higher rate (Fig. 3.32).

Always bear in mind that the P wave may be difficult or even impossible to discern clearly. Therefore, it can be difficult to say conclusively that atrial activity is absent.

Is the rhythm regular or irregular?

To determine whether the cardiac rhythm is regular, measure the distance between consecutive R waves on a rhythm strip. If the RR interval varies, the rhythm is irregular (Table 3.5).

Table 3.5 Irregular cardiac rhythms

- Sinus arrhythmia
- Atrial fibrillation
- Ventricular fibrillation
- Any supraventricular rhythm with intermittent block
- Ectopic beats

If an impulse is blocked *en route* to the ventricles as a result of a conduction disturbance, the corresponding QRS complex will fail to appear where expected and the beat will be 'missed' (Fig. 3.33), as discussed on p. 60.

Ectopic beats appear *earlier* than expected (Fig. 3.34), and are discussed on p. 63.

Is there a bradycardia or tachycardia?

The arrhythmias that cause an abnormal heart rate are discussed in Chapter 2.

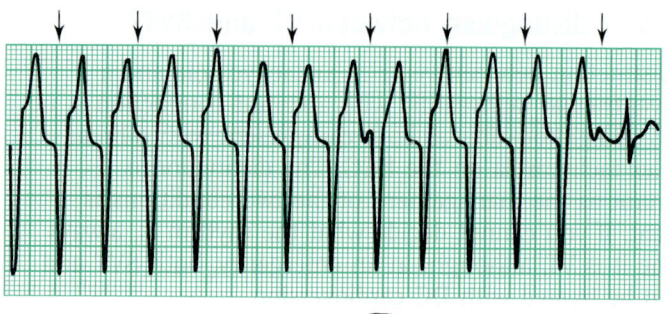

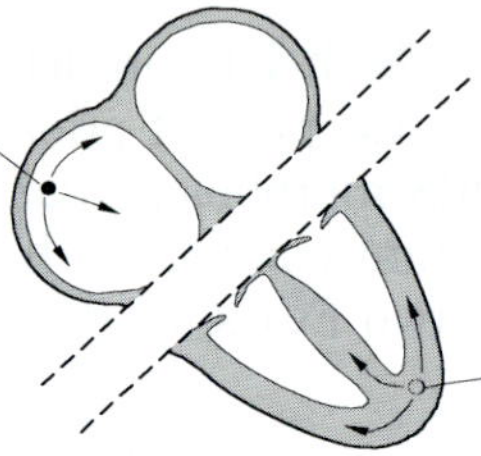

74 MAKING SENSE OF THE ECG

FIG. 3.35

Independent P wave activity

Key points:
- broad-complex tachycardia (VT)
- arrows show independent P waves deforming the QRS complexes
- last beat is a capture beat

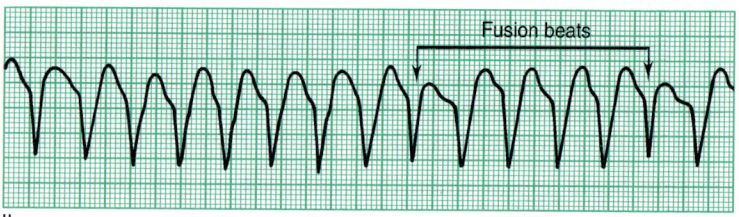

FIG. 3.36

Fusion beats

Key points:
- broad-complex tachycardia (VT)
- arrows show fusion beats

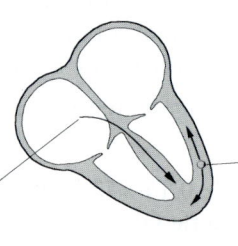

Ventricular tachycardia

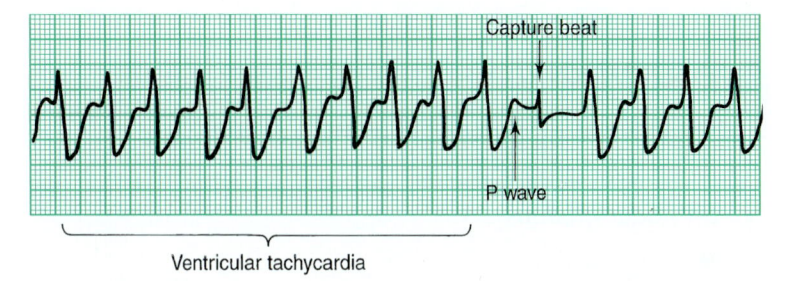

FIG. 3.37

Capture beats

Key points:
- broad-complex tachycardia
- one normal QRS complex (capture beat)

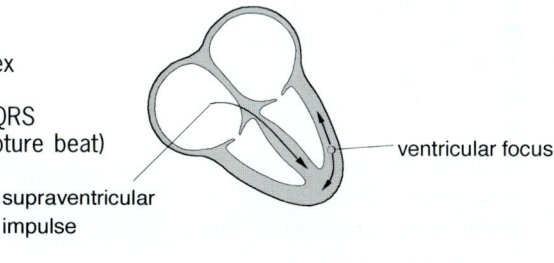

supraventricular impulse

ventricular focus

- leftward or rightward QRS axis.
- Adenosine has no effect but P waves and AV dissociation may become clearer.

If the rhythm slows or terminates with manoeuvres that slow or block conduction in the AV node, the rhythm is likely to be supraventricular with aberrant conduction.

Supraventricular tachycardia

The term 'supraventricular tachycardia' (SVT) is frequently misused and this leads to misunderstanding. Literally, it refers to any heart rate over 100 beats per minute (tachycardia) that originates above the ventricles (supraventricular). It encompasses many different arrhythmias, including sinus tachycardia, atrial fibrillation, atrial tachycardia and AV re-entry tachycardias. This is the meaning of SVT that has been used in this book. Some people use the term SVT to refer *specifically* to AV nodal re-entry tachycardias. We recommend that you identify all arrhythmias as specifically as possible, and reserve SVT as a general term for tachycardias that originate above the ventricles.

Summary

When assessing the cardiac rhythm, consider the following:

SA nodal rhythms
- Sinus rhythm
- Sinus bradycardia
- Sinus tachycardia
- Sinus arrhythmia
- Sick sinus syndrome

Atrial rhythms
- Atrial tachycardia
- Atrial flutter
- Atrial fibrillation

Atrioventricular rhythms
- AV re-entry tachycardias

Ventricular rhythms
- Ventricular tachycardia
- Accelerated idioventricular rhythm
- Torsades de pointes
- Ventricular fibrillation

Conduction disturbances
Escape rhythms
Ectopic beats

To identify the rhythm, ask the following questions:

1. Where does the impulse arise from?
- Sinoatrial (SA) node
- Atria
- Atrioventricular (AV) junction
- Ventricles

2. How is the impulse conducted?
- Normal conduction
- Accelerated conduction (e.g. WPW syndrome)
- Blocked conduction

4

THE AXIS

Working out the cardiac axis causes more confusion than almost any other aspect of ECG assessment. This should not really be the case, as there is no mystery to the cardiac axis and it is usually very straightforward to assess. Indeed, deciding whether the cardiac axis is normal can be summarized in one rule:

> **A quick rule for assessing the axis**
>
> If the QRS complexes are predominantly positive in leads I and II, then the cardiac axis is normal.

If you are confident about assessing the axis, you can go straight to the second half of this chapter, where we will explain the causes of an abnormal axis. If not, read through the first half of the chapter, where we explain in straightforward terms what the axis represents and how it can be measured.

What does the axis mean?

As we explained in Chapter 1, the flow of electrical current through the heart is fairly uniform, as it normally passes along a well-defined pathway (Fig. 4.1).

78 MAKING SENSE OF THE ECG

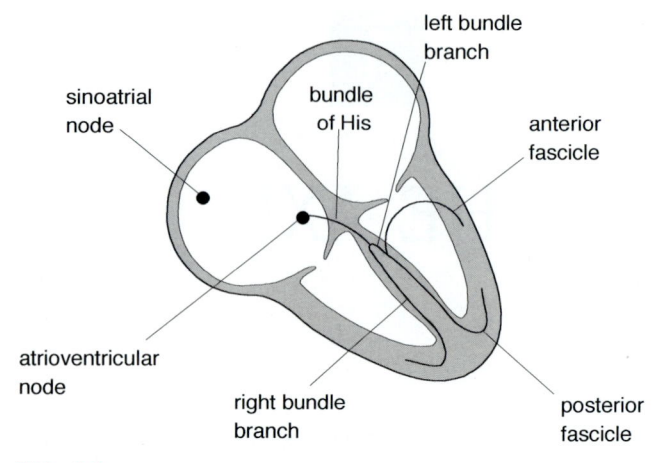

FIG. 4.1

The flow of electrical impulses through the heart

Key points:
- impulses originate in the sinoatrial node
- impulses reach the ventricles via the atrioventricular node

In simple terms, the cardiac axis is an indicator of the general direction that the wave of depolarization takes as it flows through the ventricles. If you think just about the general direction of electrical current as it flows through the ventricles, it starts at the 'top right hand corner' and flows towards the 'bottom left hand corner' (Fig. 4.2).

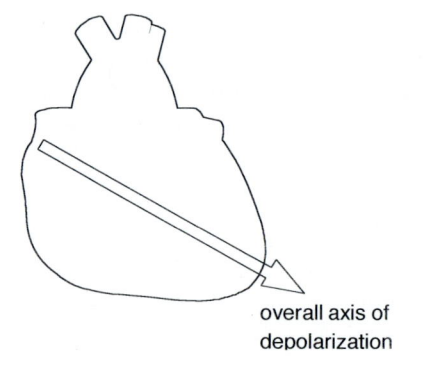

FIG. 4.2

The general direction of flow of electrical current through the heart

Key points:
- flow starts at the 'top right-hand corner'
- flow is towards the 'bottom left-hand corner'

What measurement is used for the axis?

When describing the axis, a more precise terminology is required. The axis is therefore conventionally referred to as the angle, measured in degrees, of the direction of electrical current flowing through the ventricles.

The reference, or zero, point is taken as a horizontal line 'looking' at the heart from the left (Fig. 4.3). For a direction of flow directed below the line, the angle is expressed as a positive number; above the line, as a negative number (Fig. 4.4). Thus, the cardiac axis can be either +1° to +180°, or –1° to –180°.

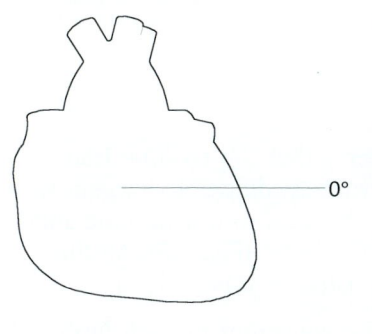

FIG. 4.3

The reference (or 'zero') point for axis measurements

Key points:
- the zero point is a horizontal line looking at the heart from the left
- this is the same as the viewpoint of lead I
- all axis measurements are made relative to this line

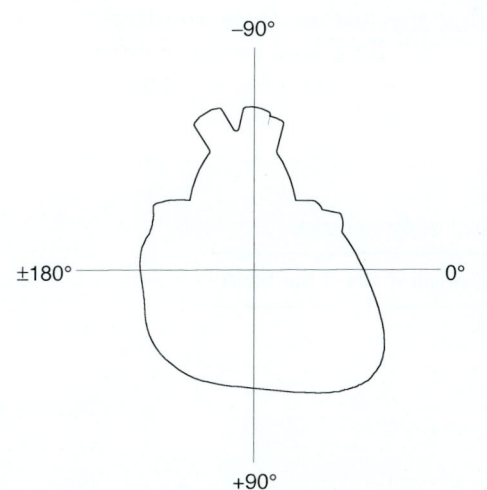

FIG. 4.4

The range of angles of the cardiac axis

Key points:
- anticlockwise measurements are negative
- clockwise measurements are positive
- all measurements are relative to the zero line

FIG. 4.5

Viewpoints of the six limb leads

Key point:
- each lead looks at the heart from a different angle

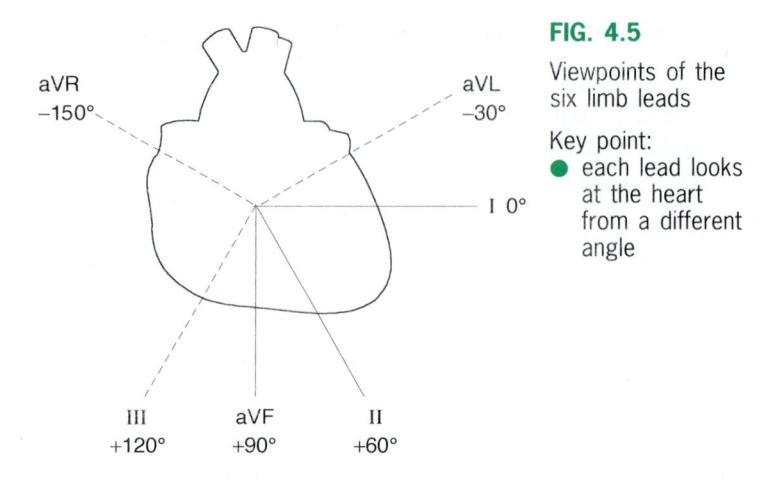

You will remember from Chapter 1 that the six limb leads look at the heart sideways on from six different viewpoints. The same reference system can be used to describe the angle from which each lead looks at the heart (Fig. 4.5). All the limb leads and their angles are listed in Table 4.1.

Make an effort to remember the viewpoint of each limb lead now, before reading any further. Once you have grasped the concept of each limb lead having a different angle of view of the heart, understanding the cardiac axis will be easy.

Table 4.1 Limb leads and angles of view

Limb lead	Angle at which it views the heart
I	0°
II	+60°
III	+120°
aVR	−150°
aVL	−30°
aVF	+90°

How do I use the limb leads to work out the axis?

The information from the limb leads is used to work out the cardiac axis. Simply remember three principles, all of which we have covered already:

- The axis is the general direction of electrical flow through the heart.
- Each of the limb leads records this electrical flow from a different viewpoint of the heart.
- Electrical flow towards a lead causes a positive deflection, and flow away from a lead causes a negative deflection.

This last rule means that if current flows at right angles to a lead, then the ECG complex generated will be isoelectric (the positive and negative deflections cancel each other out). This is illustrated in Fig. 4.6.

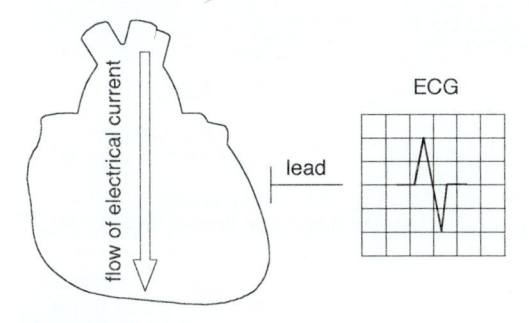

FIG. 4.6

An isoelectric ECG complex

Key point: ● current flow at right angles to a lead causes an isoelectric complex

Using these principles, consider how lead II records ventricular depolarization. From its point of view, the flow of current in the ventricles is entirely towards it and the QRS complex is entirely positive (Fig. 4.7). Lead aVL, however, will see the same current at right angles to itself and record an isoelectric QRS complex (Fig. 4.8). Any leads looking from a viewpoint

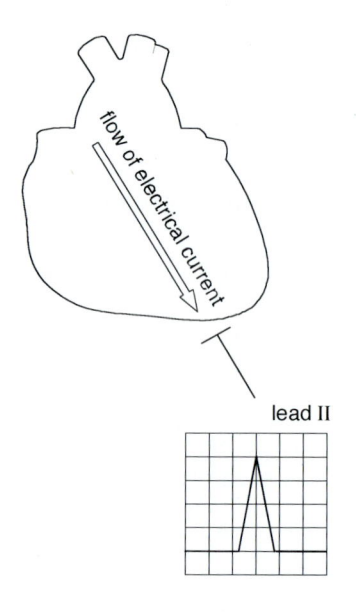

FIG. 4.7

The QRS complex is entirely positive in lead II

Key points:
- flow towards a lead causes a positive deflection
- current flow in the ventricles is towards lead II

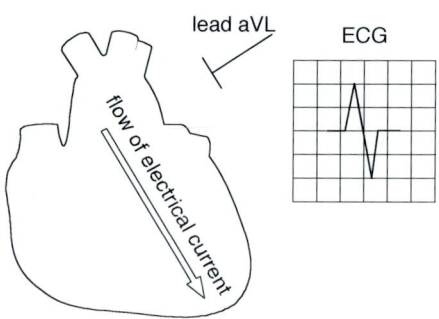

FIG. 4.8

The QRS complex is isoelectric in lead aVL

Key points:
- flow at right angles to a lead causes an isoelectric complex
- current flow in the ventricles is at right angles to lead aVL

between leads II and aVL will record a complex that becomes increasingly positive the closer it is to lead II (Fig. 4.9).

It should now be fairly clear that you can work out the cardiac axis by examining whether the QRS complexes in the limb leads are predominantly positive or negative.

There are two ways of determining the cardiac axis: one is quick and approximate, the other is precise but detailed.

FIG. 4.9

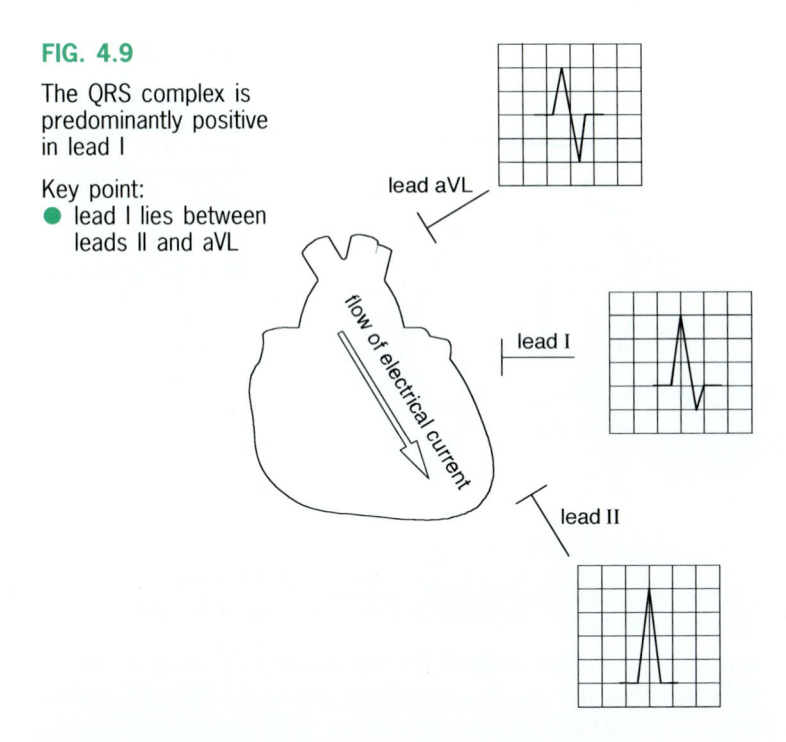

The QRS complex is predominantly positive in lead I

Key point:
- lead I lies between leads II and aVL

A quick way to work out the cardiac axis

This technique enables you to decide within seconds whether the axis is normal or abnormal. To decide if the axis is normal, you need only look at two of the limb leads: I and II.

What is a 'normal' axis?

Unfortunately, there is not universal agreement on what is a normal axis. For the purposes of this book, we consider a normal axis to be anything between −30° and +90°, although we should mention that some cardiologists accept anything up to +120° as normal. This is because there is no definitive dividing line between normality and abnormality. The most sensible approach is to consider that the *likelihood* of a patient having an underlying abnormality increases as the axis increases from +90° to +120°.

FIG. 4.10

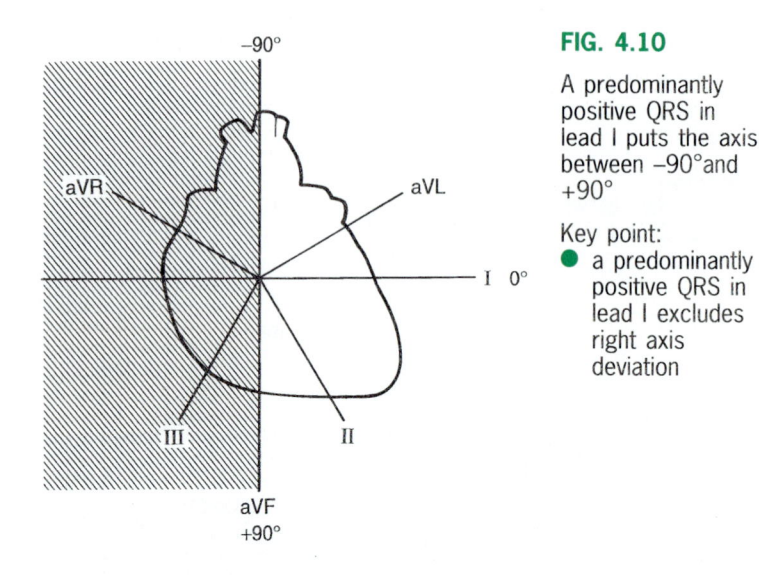

A predominantly positive QRS in lead I puts the axis between −90° and +90°

Key point:
- a predominantly positive QRS in lead I excludes right axis deviation

If the QRS complex in **lead I** is predominantly positive, this indicates that the axis lies anywhere between −90° and +90° (Fig. 4.10). An axis at *exactly* −90° or +90° would cause a precisely isoelectric QRS complex in lead I. Thus, a predominantly positive QRS complex in lead I rules out right axis deviation (an axis beyond +90°), but does not exclude left axis deviation (an axis beyond −30°).

If the QRS complex in **lead II** is predominantly positive, this indicates that the axis lies anywhere between −30° and +150° (Fig. 4.11). An axis at *exactly* −30° or +150° would cause a precisely isoelectric QRS complex in lead II. Thus, a predominantly positive QRS complex in lead II rules out left axis deviation (an axis beyond −30°), but does not exclude right axis deviation (an axis beyond +90°).

However, by looking at whether the QRS complex is positive or negative in both these leads, it is possible to say immediately whether the axis is normal, or whether there is left or right axis deviation:

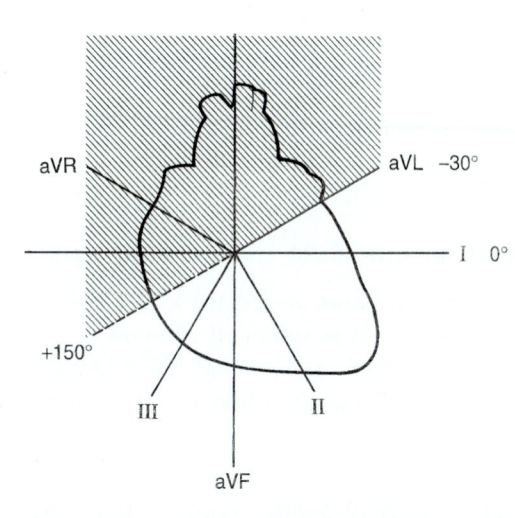

FIG. 4.11

A predominantly positive QRS in lead II puts the axis between −30° and +150°

Key point:
- a predominantly positive QRS in lead II excludes left axis deviation

- A predominantly positive QRS complex in both leads I and II means the **axis is normal**.
- A predominantly positive QRS complex in lead I and predominantly negative QRS complex in lead II means there is **left axis deviation**.
- A predominantly negative QRS complex in lead I and predominantly positive QRS complex in lead II means there is **right axis deviation**.

These rules are summarized in Table 4.2.

Table 4.2 Working out the cardiac axis

Lead I	Lead II	Cardiac axis
Positive QRS	Positive QRS	Normal axis
Positive QRS	Negative QRS	Left axis deviation
Negative QRS	Positive QRS	Right axis deviation

When you assess the cardiac axis you should therefore ask the following questions:

- Is there left axis deviation?
- Is there right axis deviation?

The causes of these abnormalities, with guidance on their management, are discussed in the second half of this chapter.

A more precise way to calculate the cardiac axis

For most practical purposes, it is not necessary to determine precisely the axis of the heart – it is sufficient to know simply whether the axis is normal or abnormal. Calculating the axis precisely is not difficult but does take a little time – this section explains how.

The method relies upon the use of vectors and a knowledge of how to calculate angles in right-angled triangles. Begin by finding two leads that look at the heart at right angles to each other, for example leads I and aVF (Fig. 4.12).

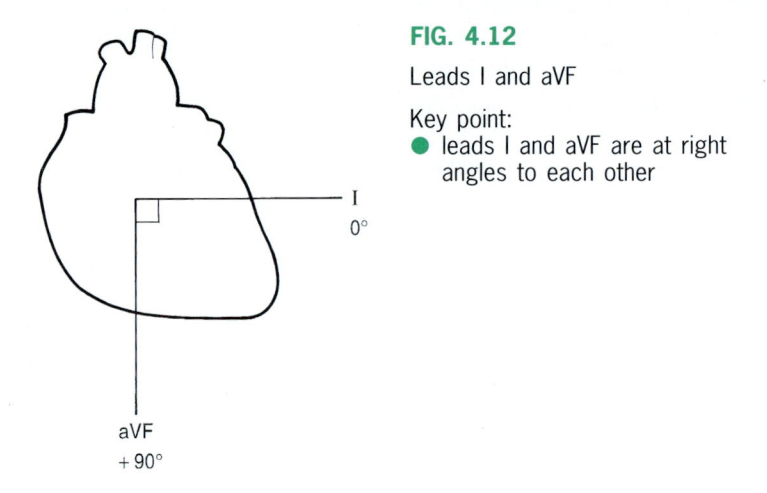

FIG. 4.12

Leads I and aVF

Key point:
- leads I and aVF are at right angles to each other

Look at the QRS complexes in these leads, and work out their overall sizes and polarities by subtracting the depth of the S wave from the height of the R wave (Fig. 4.13). The

THE AXIS 87

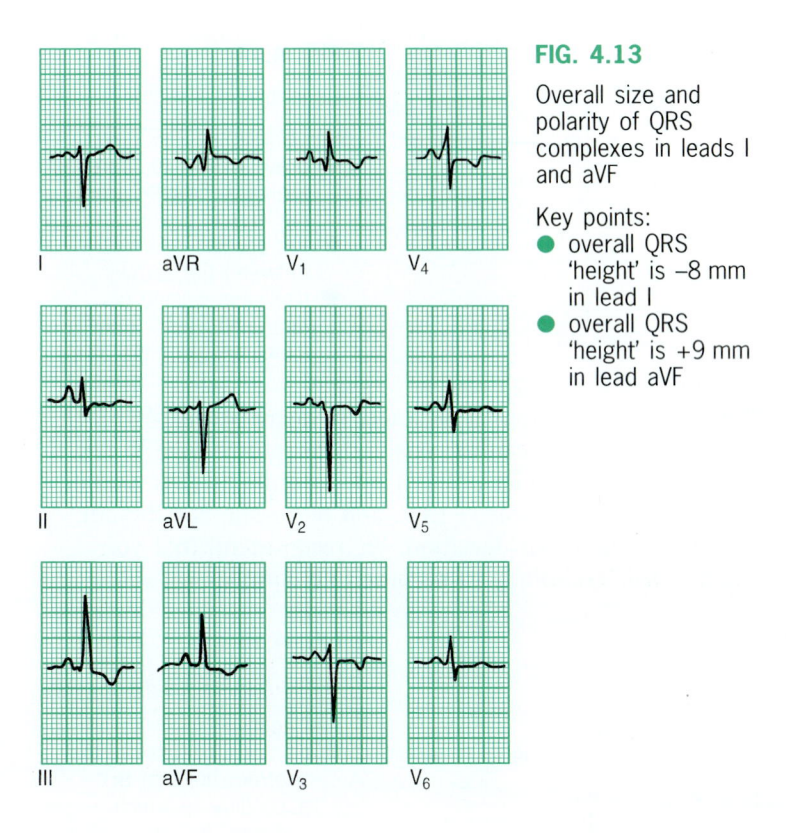

FIG. 4.13

Overall size and polarity of QRS complexes in leads I and aVF

Key points:
- overall QRS 'height' is −8 mm in lead I
- overall QRS 'height' is +9 mm in lead aVF

polarity (positive or negative) tells you whether the impulse is moving towards or away from the lead. The overall size tells you how much of the electricity is flowing in that direction. Using this information, you can construct a vector diagram (Fig. 4.14).

Thus, by combining the information from the two leads, you can use a pocket calculator to work out the angle at which the current is flowing (i.e. the cardiac axis). Remember:

- sine of an angle = opposite edge/hypotenuse
- cosine of an angle = adjacent edge/hypotenuse
- tangent of an angle = opposite edge/adjacent edge

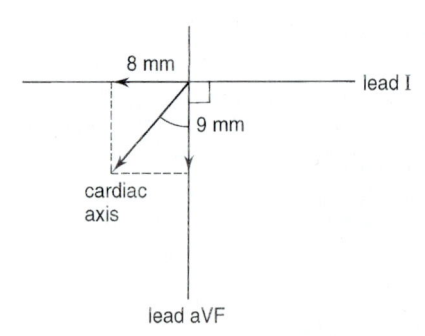

FIG. 4.14

Constructing a vector diagram

Key points:
- draw arrows to represent the QRS 'heights' from Fig. 4.13
- the cardiac axis lies between the arrows
- use sine, cosine or tangent to work out the exact angle of the axis

Thus, we finally arrive at an angle in degrees (Fig. 4.15). Do not forget that the cardiac axis is measured relative to lead I, and to add or subtract units of 90° accordingly. The axis in this patient is therefore +132°, and he or she has (by our definition) right axis deviation. We recommend that you practise this technique to become fully familiar with it.

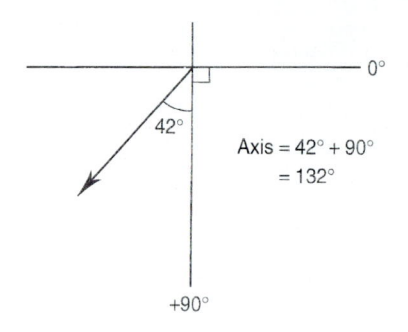

FIG. 4.15

Working out the cardiac axis

Key point:
- do not forget to add or subtract units of 90° according to which quadrant the axis lies in

P and T wave axes

So far, we have concentrated on the axis of depolarization as it flows through the ventricles, and this is generally referred to as the cardiac axis. However, it is also possible to work out an axis for atrial depolarization (by applying the vector analysis we have described to P waves) and for ventricular repolarization (using T waves). These measurements are seldom necessary, except where a more detailed analysis of the ECG is required.

IS THERE LEFT AXIS DEVIATION?

Left axis deviation is present when the cardiac axis lies beyond −30°. This sometimes occurs in normal individuals, but more often indicates one of the following:

- left anterior hemiblock
- Wolff–Parkinson–White syndrome
- inferior myocardial infarction
- ventricular tachycardia.

These are discussed on the following pages.

Left ventricular hypertrophy can cause left axis deviation but *not* as a result of increased muscle mass (unlike right ventricular hypertrophy). Instead, it results from left anterior hemiblock caused by fibrosis. Contrary to some textbooks, neither obesity nor pregnancy cause left axis deviation (although obesity *can* cause a leftward shift with the axis staying within normal limits).

Left anterior hemiblock

In Chapter 1, we described how electrical impulses are conducted within the interventricular septum in the left and right bundle branches, and that the left bundle branch divides into anterior and posterior fascicles (Fig. 1.16). Either (or both) of these fascicles can be blocked. Block of the left anterior fascicle is called left anterior hemiblock, and is the commonest cause of left axis deviation (Fig. 4.16).

Left anterior hemiblock can occur as a result of fibrosis of the conducting system (of any cause), or from myocardial infarction. On its own, it is not thought to carry any prognostic significance. However, left anterior hemiblock in combination with right bundle branch block (p. 144) means that two of the three main conducting pathways to the ventricles are blocked. This is termed **bifascicular** block (Fig. 4.17).

FIG. 4.16

Left axis deviation

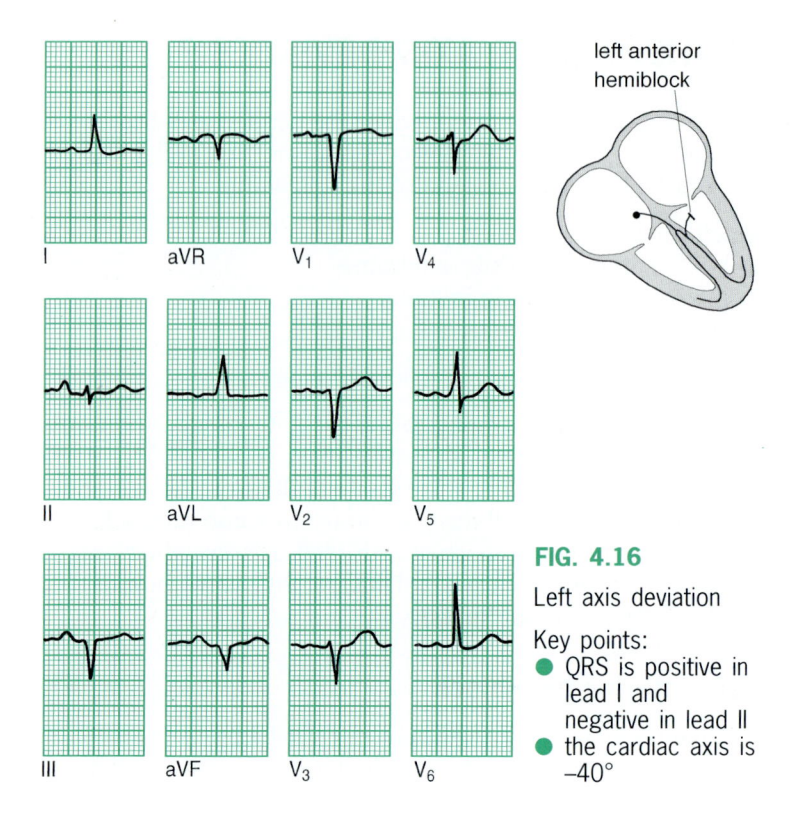

Key points:
- QRS is positive in lead I and negative in lead II
- the cardiac axis is −40°

Block of the conducting pathways can occur in any combination. A block of both fascicles is the equivalent of left bundle branch block. Block of the right bundle branch and either fascicle is bifascicular block. If bifascicular block is combined with first-degree AV block (long PR interval), this is called **trifascicular** block (Fig. 4.18). Block of the right bundle branch and both fascicles leaves no route for impulses to reach the ventricles, and this is the equivalent of third-degree ('complete') AV block.

Bifascicular block in a patient with syncopal episodes is often sufficient indication for a permanent pacemaker, even if higher degrees of block have not been documented. Referral

FIG. 4.17

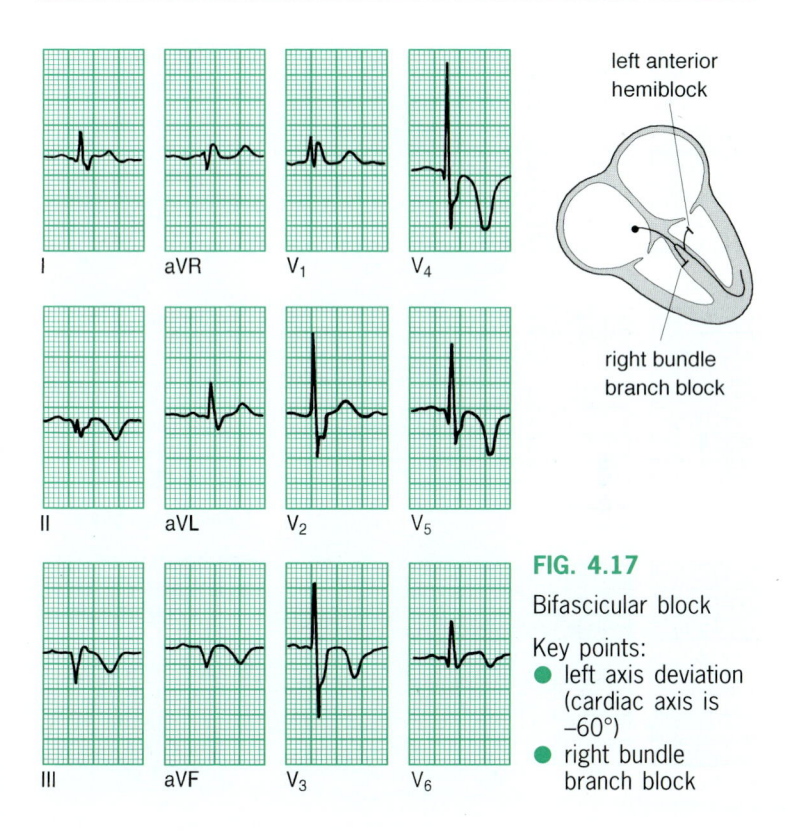

Bifascicular block

Key points:
- left axis deviation (cardiac axis is −60°)
- right bundle branch block

of these patients to a cardiologist is therefore recommended. *Asymptomatic* bifascicular block, or even trifascicular block, is not necessarily an indication for pacing – discuss with a cardiologist if in doubt.

SEEK HELP

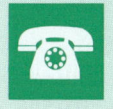

Bifascicular block with syncope usually requires pacing. Referral to a cardiologist is recommended.

FIG. 4.18

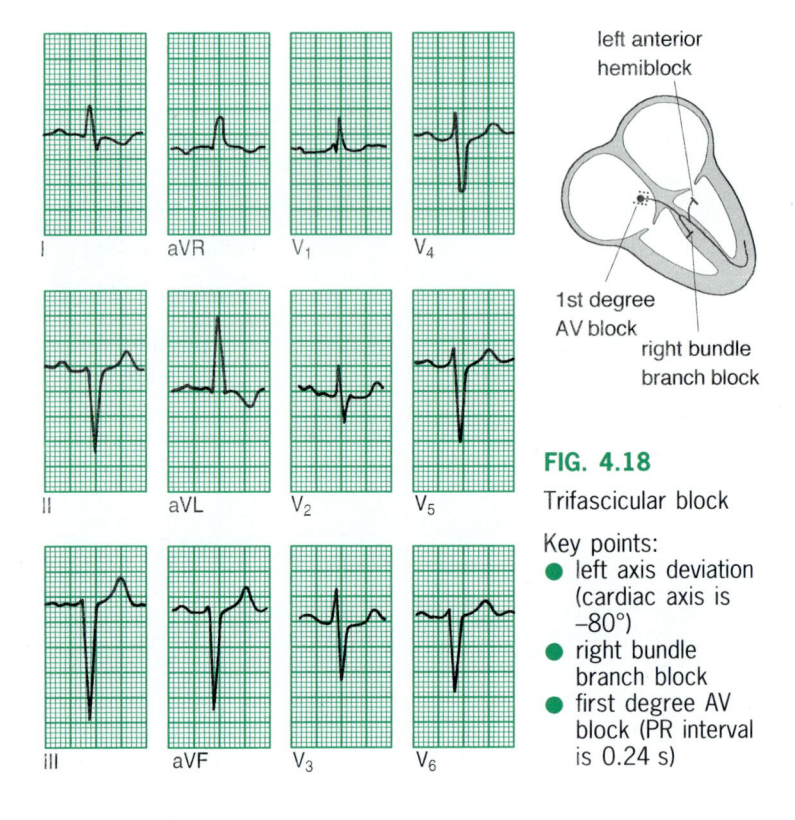

Trifascicular block

Key points:
- left axis deviation (cardiac axis is −80°)
- right bundle branch block
- first degree AV block (PR interval is 0.24 s)

Wolff–Parkinson–White syndrome

Patients with Wolff–Parkinson–White (WPW) syndrome have an accessory pathway that bypasses the AV node and bundle of His to connect the atria directly to the ventricles. If this pathway lies between the atria and ventricles on the right side of the heart, patients may have left axis deviation in addition to the other ECG appearances of WPW syndrome. The management of WPW syndrome is discussed on p. 111.

Inferior myocardial infarction

Left axis deviation may be a feature of myocardial infarction affecting the inferior aspect of the heart (the cardiac axis is directed away from infarcted areas). The diagnosis will usually be apparent from the presentation and other ECG findings. For more information on the diagnosis and treatment of acute myocardial infarction, turn to p. 156.

Ventricular tachycardia (with LV apical focus)

When ventricular tachycardia arises from a focus in the left ventricle, the wave of depolarization spreads out through the rest of the myocardium from that point, resulting in left axis deviation. The diagnosis and treatment of ventricular tachycardia is discussed on p. 55.

IS THERE RIGHT AXIS DEVIATION?

Right axis deviation is present when the cardiac axis lies beyond +90°. This sometimes occurs in normal individuals, but more often indicates one of the following:

- right ventricular hypertrophy
- Wolff–Parkinson–White syndrome
- anterolateral myocardial infarction
- dextrocardia
- left posterior hemiblock.

These are discussed on the following pages.

Right ventricular hypertrophy

Right ventricular hypertrophy is the commonest cause of right axis deviation (Fig. 4.19).

Other ECG evidence of right ventricular hypertrophy includes:

- dominant R wave in lead V_1
- deep S waves in leads V_5 and V_6
- right bundle branch block.

For more information on the causes of right ventricular hypertrophy, turn to p. 136.

Summary

To assess the cardiac axis, ask the following questions:

1. Is there left axis deviation?

If 'yes', consider:

- Left anterior hemiblock
- Wolff–Parkinson–White syndrome
- Inferior myocardial infarction
- Ventricular tachycardia (with LV apical focus)

2. Is there right axis deviation?

If 'yes', consider:

- Right ventricular hypertrophy
- Wolff–Parkinson–White syndrome
- Anterolateral myocardial infarction
- Dextrocardia
- Left posterior hemiblock

5

THE P WAVE

After determining the heart rate, rhythm and axis, you should examine each wave of the ECG in turn, beginning with the P wave. You may already have noticed abnormal P waves while assessing the cardiac rhythm, but in this chapter we will tell you how to examine the P wave in more detail and what abnormalities to look out for.

As you examine the P wave in each lead, the questions to ask are:

- Are any P waves absent?
- Are any P waves inverted?
- Are any P waves too tall?
- Are any P waves too wide?

In this chapter, we will help you to answer these questions and to interpret any abnormalities you may find.

The origin of the P wave

You will recall from Chapter 1 that the P wave represents **atrial depolarization**. It does not, as some people mistakenly believe, represent *SA node* depolarization; it is possible to have P waves without SA node depolarization (e.g. atrial ectopics), or SA node depolarization without P waves (sinoatrial block).

ARE ANY P WAVES ABSENT?

The sinoatrial node is normally a very regular and dependable natural pacemaker. Atrial depolarization, and thus P wave formation, is therefore normally so regular that it is easy to predict when the next P wave is going to appear (Fig. 5.1).

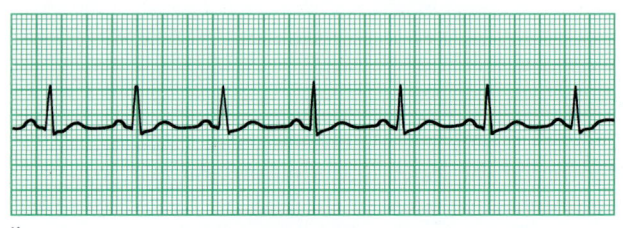

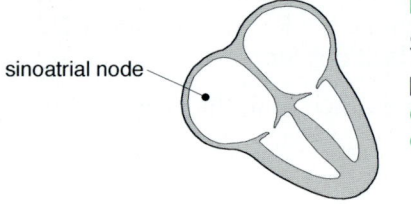

FIG. 5.1

Sinus rhythm

Key points:
- regular P waves
- it is easy to predict when the next P wave will appear

The only normal circumstance in which the P wave rate is variable is sinus arrhythmia, which is usually only seen in patients below the age of 40 years. Sinus arrhythmia was discussed on p. 37.

In this section, we will tell you what diagnoses to consider if you find that P waves are absent. By this, we mean that they can be either:

- completely absent (no P waves on the whole ECG)

or:

- intermittently absent (some P waves do not appear where expected).

P waves are completely absent

There are two reasons why P waves may be absent from the ECG. The first is that there is no co-ordinated atrial activity so that P waves are not being formed. The second is that P waves *are* present, but are just not obvious.

A lack of co-ordinated atrial activity occurs in **atrial fibrillation**, and this is the commonest reason for P waves to be truly absent from the ECG (Fig. 5.2). Instead of P waves, the chaotic atrial activity produces low-amplitude oscillations (fibrillation or 'f' waves) on the ECG. Atrial fibrillation can be recognized by the absence of P waves and the erratic formation of QRS complexes. The causes and treatment of atrial fibrillation are discussed on p. 44.

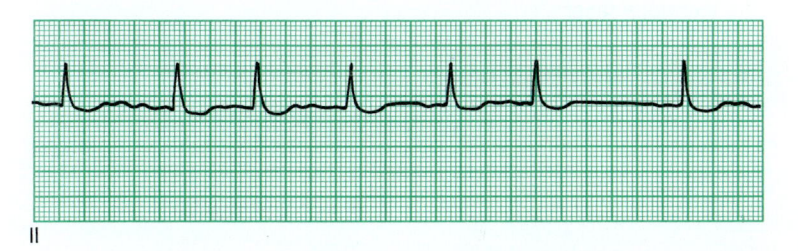

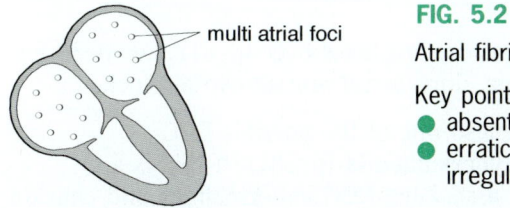

FIG. 5.2
Atrial fibrillation

Key points:
- absent P waves
- erratic ('irregularly irregular') QRS rhythm

P waves will also be completely absent if there is a prolonged period of **sinus arrest** or **sinoatrial block** (Fig. 5.3). In these conditions, atrial activation does not occur because the SA node either fails to depolarize (sinus arrest) or fails to transmit the depolarization to the atria (sinoatrial block). Either condition *can* cause ventricular asystole, but more

FIG. 5.3

Sinus arrest

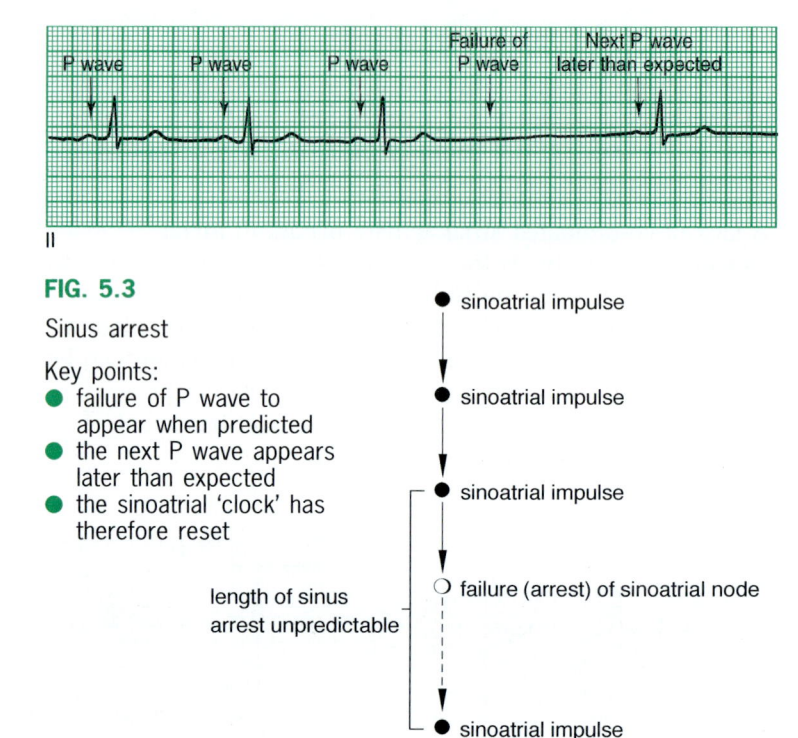

Key points:
- failure of P wave to appear when predicted
- the next P wave appears later than expected
- the sinoatrial 'clock' has therefore reset

commonly an escape rhythm takes over (p. 61). See p. 38 for more information on sinus arrest and sinoatrial block.

Absent P waves are also one of the possible ECG manifestations of **hyperkalaemia** (p. 181). If this is a possibility, look for associated ECG abnormalities and check a plasma potassium level urgently.

It is very common for P waves to be present but not immediately obvious. Search the ECG carefully for evidence of P waves before concluding that they are absent, as P waves will often be hidden by **any rapid tachycardia**. Figure 5.4 shows an AV junctional tachycardia with a heart rate of 130 beats per minute. At first glance, the P waves appear to

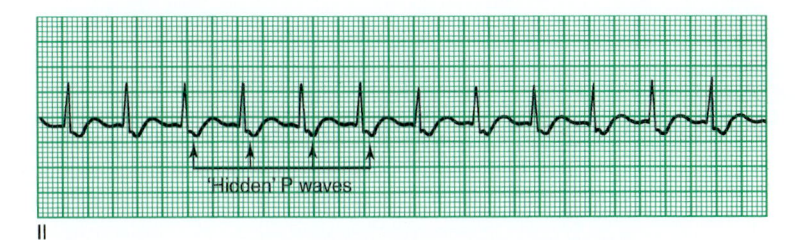

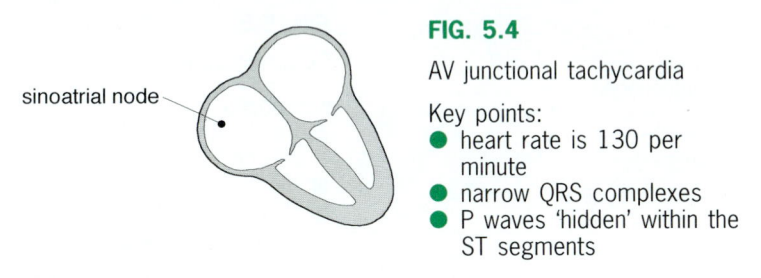

FIG. 5.4

AV junctional tachycardia

Key points:
- heart rate is 130 per minute
- narrow QRS complexes
- P waves 'hidden' within the ST segments

be absent. On closer inspection, they can just be seen buried within the ST segments.

Even in sinus tachycardia, at high heart rates the P wave may start to overlap with the T wave of the previous beat, making it hard to identify (Fig. 5.5).

At very high atrial rates, such as in atrial flutter, P waves may not be apparent because they become distorted. In atrial flutter, the atria usually depolarize around 300 times per minute. The P waves generated by this rapid activity are called flutter waves, and have a 'sawtooth' appearance. Atrial flutter is discussed on p. 42.

In ventricular tachycardia, retrograde (backward) conduction up through the AV node may cause each ventricular complex to be *followed* by a P wave which may not be immediately obvious and which also, incidentally, will be inverted. Even more importantly, *independent* atrial activity can occur during ventricular tachycardia, and the P waves can be buried anywhere within the QRS complexes (Fig. 3.35). Evidence of independent atrial activity is a very useful clue

FIG. 5.5

Sinus tachycardia

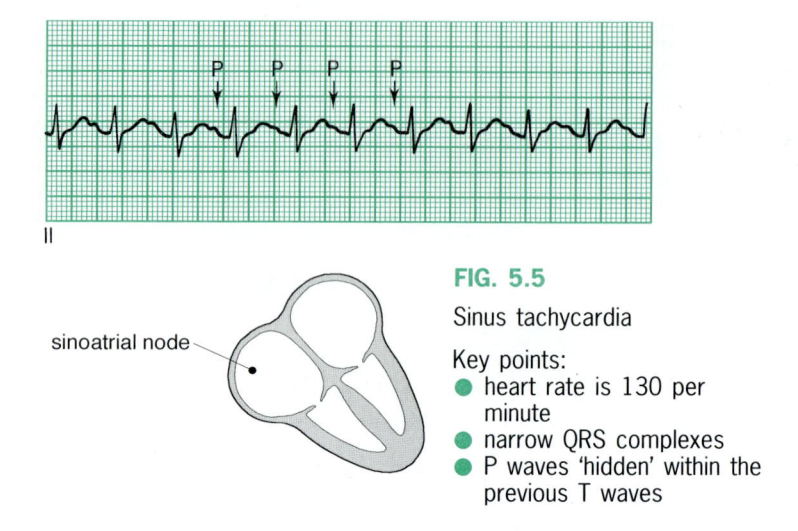

Key points:
- heart rate is 130 per minute
- narrow QRS complexes
- P waves 'hidden' within the previous T waves

in the differentiation of ventricular and supraventricular tachycardias.

More information about all of these cardiac rhythms can be found in Chapter 3.

P waves are intermittently absent

The SA node is usually an extremely reliable natural pacemaker. The occasional absence of a P wave on an ECG indicates that the SA node has either failed to generate an impulse (sinus arrest), or failed to conduct the impulse to the surrounding atrial tissue (sinoatrial block).

For examples of both these conditions, together with guidance on how to distinguish them, turn to p. 38.

ARE ANY P WAVES INVERTED?

The P wave is usually upright in all leads except aVR, which 'looks' at the atria from roughly the patient's right shoulder and so detects the wave of atrial depolarization moving away

FIG. 5.6

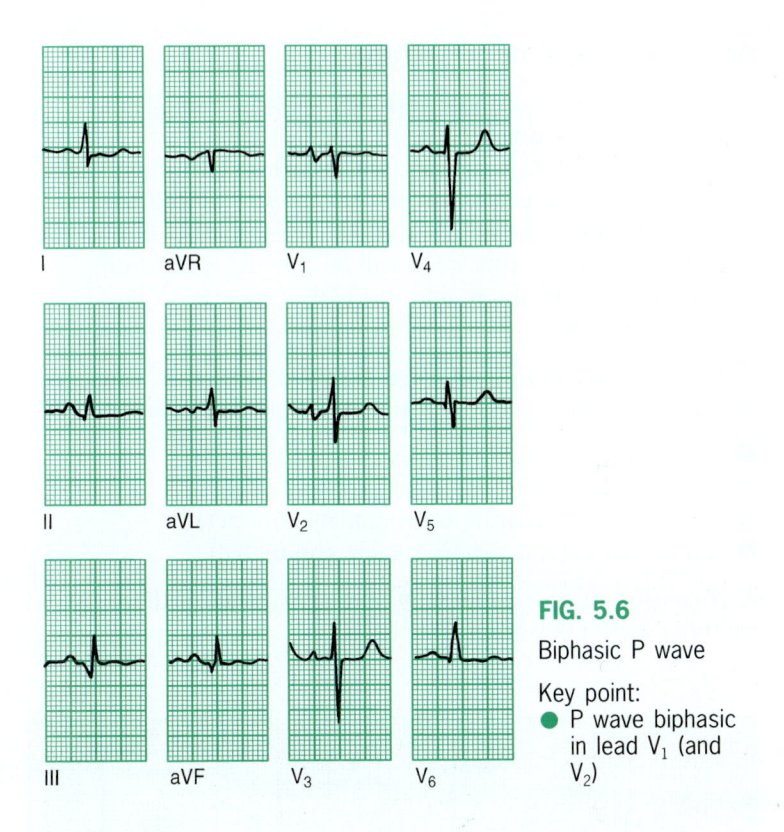

Biphasic P wave

Key point:
- P wave biphasic in lead V_1 (and V_2)

from it (Fig. 1.8). The P wave may sometimes be inverted in lead V_1 also, although it is more usually biphasic in that lead (Fig. 5.6).

Whenever you see an inverted P wave, ask yourself:

- Were the electrodes correctly positioned?

Abnormal P wave inversion can indicate either of the following:

- dextrocardia
- abnormal atrial depolarization.

Dextrocardia is discussed on p. 139. Abnormal atrial depolarization is explained on p. 104.

Abnormal atrial depolarization

The wave of depolarization normally spreads through the atria from the SA node to the AV node. If atrial depolarization is initiated from within, near or through the AV node, the wave will travel in the opposite (retrograde) direction through the atria. From the 'viewpoints' of most of the ECG electrodes, this wave will be moving *away from* rather than toward them, and *inverted* P waves will be produced (Fig. 5.7).

Many abnormal sources of atrial activation can thus cause retrograde depolarization and inverted P waves, including:

- atrial ectopics
- AV junctional rhythms
- ventricular tachycardia (retrogradely conducted)
- ventricular ectopics (retrogradely conducted).

A discussion of how to identify and manage all of these rhythms can be found in Chapter 3.

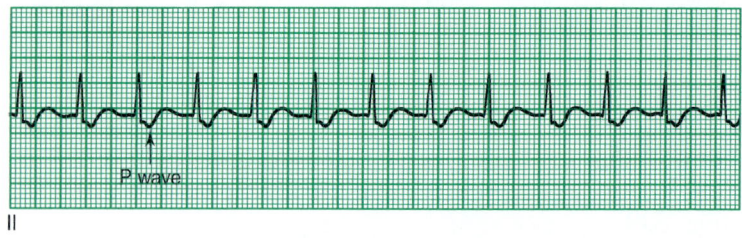

FIG. 5.7

AV junctional tachycardia

Key points:
- heart rate 130 per minute
- P waves follow QRS complexes
- P waves inverted in lead II

ARE ANY P WAVES TOO TALL?

Tall, peaked P waves indicate right atrial enlargement. The abnormality is sometimes referred to as 'P pulmonale', because right atrial enlargement is often secondary to pulmonary disorders. There is no clear 'normal range' for P wave height, but any P wave over 2.5 mm (2.5 small squares) in height should arouse suspicion. An example is shown in Fig. 5.8.

If the P waves appear unusually tall, assess your patient for any of the causes of right atrial enlargement (Table 5.1).

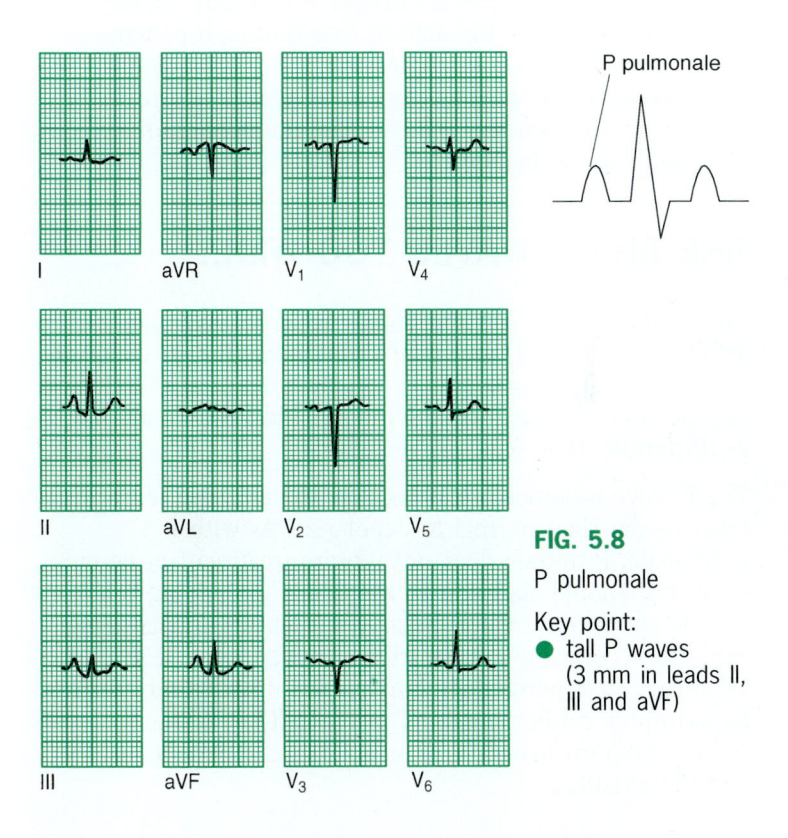

FIG. 5.8

P pulmonale

Key point:
- tall P waves (3 mm in leads II, III and aVF)

Table 5.1 Causes of right atrial enlargement

- Primary pulmonary hypertension
- Secondary pulmonary hypertension
  - chronic bronchitis
  - emphysema
  - massive pulmonary embolism
- Pulmonary stenosis
- Tricuspid stenosis

Abnormally tall P waves should draw attention to the possibility of an underlying disorder which may require further investigation. In addition to a thorough patient history and examination, a chest X-ray (to assess cardiac dimensions and lung fields) and an echocardiogram (to assess valvular disorders and estimate pulmonary artery pressure) may be helpful.

ARE ANY P WAVES TOO WIDE?

Any P waves which are abnormally wide (> 0.08 s, or 2 small squares across) and bifid should raise the suspicion of left atrial enlargement. This is usually a result of mitral valve disease, and consequently the broad, bifid P waves are known as 'P mitrale' (Fig. 5.9).

The P wave becomes broad because the enlarged left atrium takes longer than normal to depolarize. As with P pulmonale, P mitrale does not require treatment in its own right, but should alert you to a possible underlying problem. This is often mitral valve disease, but left atrial enlargement can also accompany left ventricular hypertrophy (e.g. secondary to hypertension, aortic valve disease and hypertrophic cardiomyopathy). A chest X-ray and an echocardiogram may be helpful following a patient history and examination.

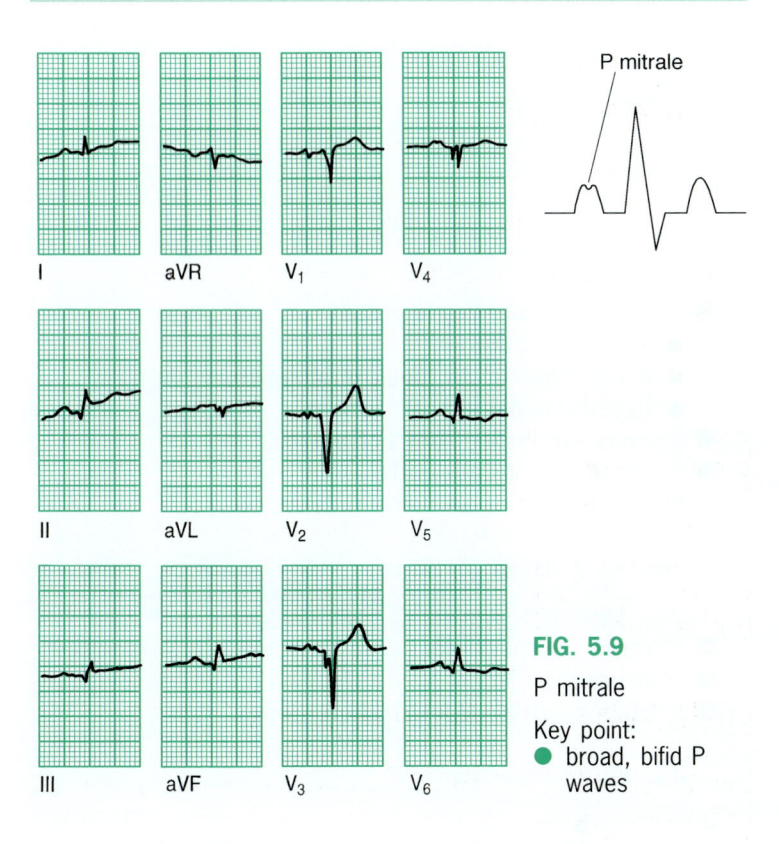

THE P WAVE

FIG. 5.9

P mitrale

Key point:
- broad, bifid P waves

Summary

To assess the P wave, ask the following questions:

1. Are any P waves absent?

If 'yes', consider:
- P waves are completely absent
  - atrial fibrillation
  - sinus arrest or SA block (prolonged)
  - hyperkalaemia
- P waves are present but not obvious
- P waves are intermittently absent
  - sinus arrest or SA block (intermittent)

2. Are any P waves inverted?

If 'yes', consider:
- Electrode misplacement
- Dextrocardia
- Retrograde atrial depolarization

3. Are any P waves too tall?

If 'yes', consider:
- Right atrial enlargement

4. Are any P waves too wide?

If 'yes', consider:
- Left atrial enlargement

6

THE PR INTERVAL

Once the sinus node has generated an electrical stimulus, this must be transmitted through the atria, atrioventricular (AV) node and bundle of His to reach the ventricles and bring about cardiac contraction. The time taken for this to happen is mainly taken up by the passage of the electrical impulse through the AV node, which acts as a regulator of conduction. This corresponds to the PR interval on the ECG (Fig. 6.1).

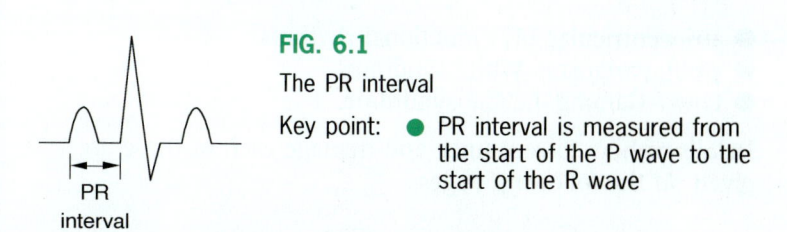

FIG. 6.1

The PR interval

Key point: ● PR interval is measured from the start of the P wave to the start of the R wave

The PR interval has precise time limits. In health, this interval is:

- no less than 0.12 s (3 small squares) long
- no more than 0.2 s (5 small squares) long
- consistent in length.

Make sure you check the duration of as many consecutive PR intervals as you can and ask the following questions:

- Is the PR interval less than 0.12 s long?
- Is the PR interval more than 0.2 s long?
- Does the PR interval vary or it cannot be measured?

This chapter will help you to answer these questions and to reach a diagnosis if you find any abnormalities.

IS THE PR INTERVAL LESS THAN 0.12 SECONDS LONG?

A PR interval of less than 0.12 s (3 small squares) indicates that the usual delay to conduction between the atria and the ventricles, imposed by the AV junction, has not occurred. This happens if depolarization *originates* in the AV junction, so that it travels up to the atria and down to the ventricles simultaneously, or if it originates as normal in the sinus node but bypasses the AV junction via an *additional faster-conducting pathway*.

A short PR interval should therefore prompt you to think of:

- atrioventricular (AV) junctional rhythms
- Wolff–Parkinson–White syndrome
- Lown–Ganong–Levine syndrome.

Details of how to recognize and manage each of these are given on the following pages.

Atrioventricular junctional rhythms

If depolarization is initiated from within the atrioventricular (AV) junction, the wave of atrial depolarization will travel backwards through the atria at the same time as setting off forwards through the AV junction towards the ventricles. Thus, the time delay between atrial depolarization (the P wave) and ventricular depolarization (the QRS complex) will be reduced (Fig. 6.2).

FIG. 6.2

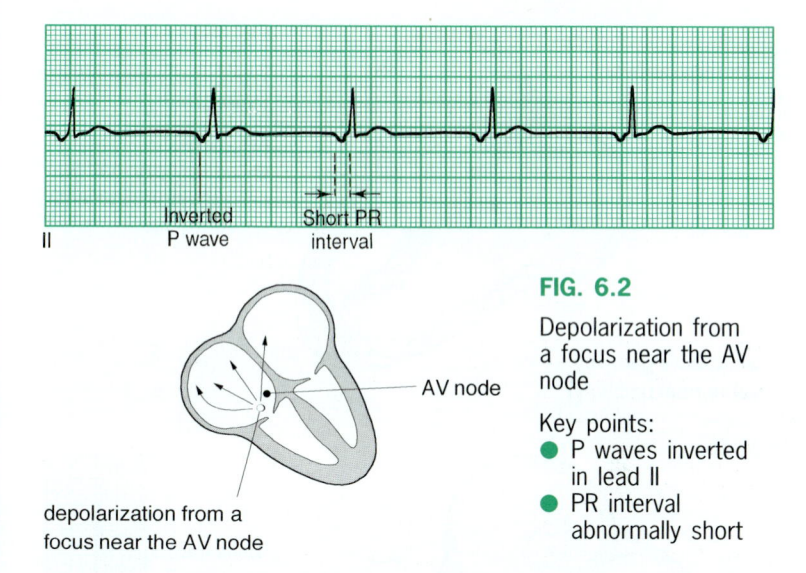

Depolarization from a focus near the AV node

Key points:
- P waves inverted in lead II
- PR interval abnormally short

Any source of depolarization within the AV junction can therefore cause a short PR interval, including:

- AV junctional escape rhythms
- AV junctional ectopics
- AV re-entry tachycardia.

A discussion of how to identify and manage all of these rhythms can be found in Chapter 3. Atrial ectopics arising near to the AV node will also have a shorter PR interval than normal sinus beats, but it will rarely be less than 0.12 s long.

Wolff–Parkinson–White syndrome

In most people, conduction of electricity through the heart follows just one distinct path from atria to ventricles; namely, via the AV node, bundle of His and the Purkinje fibres. Some people have an additional connection between the atria and the ventricles – this is Wolff–Parkinson–White (WPW) syndrome (Fig. 6.3).

FIG. 6.3

Wolff–Parkinson–White syndrome

Key point:
- accessory pathway between atria and ventricles

atrioventricular node (normal pathway)

accessory pathway (abnormal pathway)

Delta wave

accessory pathway

activated ventricle (gives rise to delta wave)

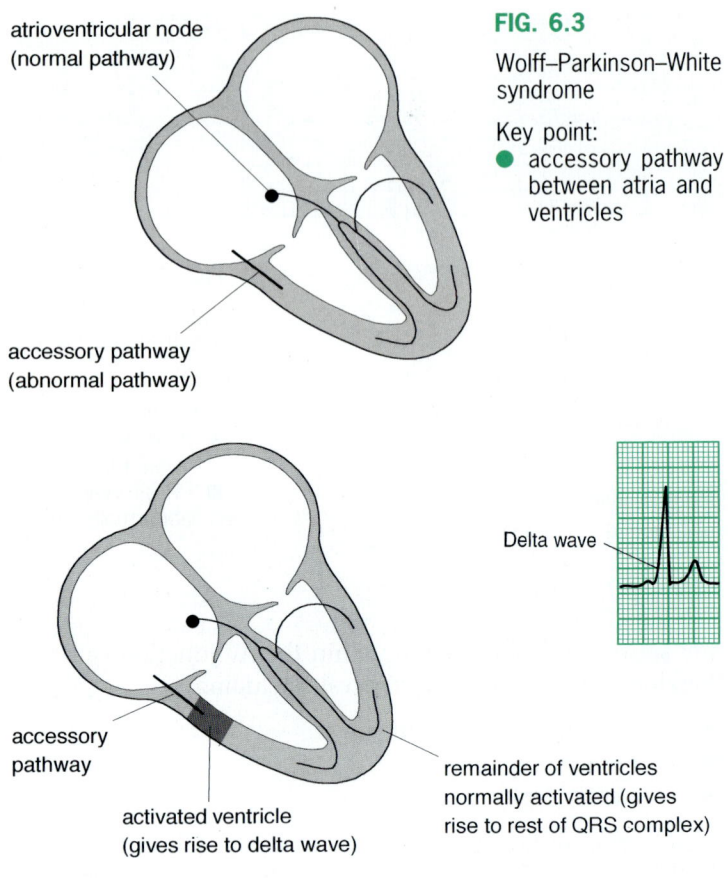

remainder of ventricles normally activated (gives rise to rest of QRS complex)

FIG. 6.4

Delta wave

Key point:
- the slurred upstroke of the QRS complex is the delta wave

The accessory pathway (called the bundle of Kent) conducts more quickly than the AV node, so the wave of depolarization reaches the ventricles more quickly than usual and thus the PR interval is short. The region of ventricle activated via the accessory pathway slowly depolarizes, giving

THE PR INTERVAL

FIG. 6.5

Wolff–Parkinson–White syndrome

Key points:
- short PR interval (0.08 s)
- delta wave

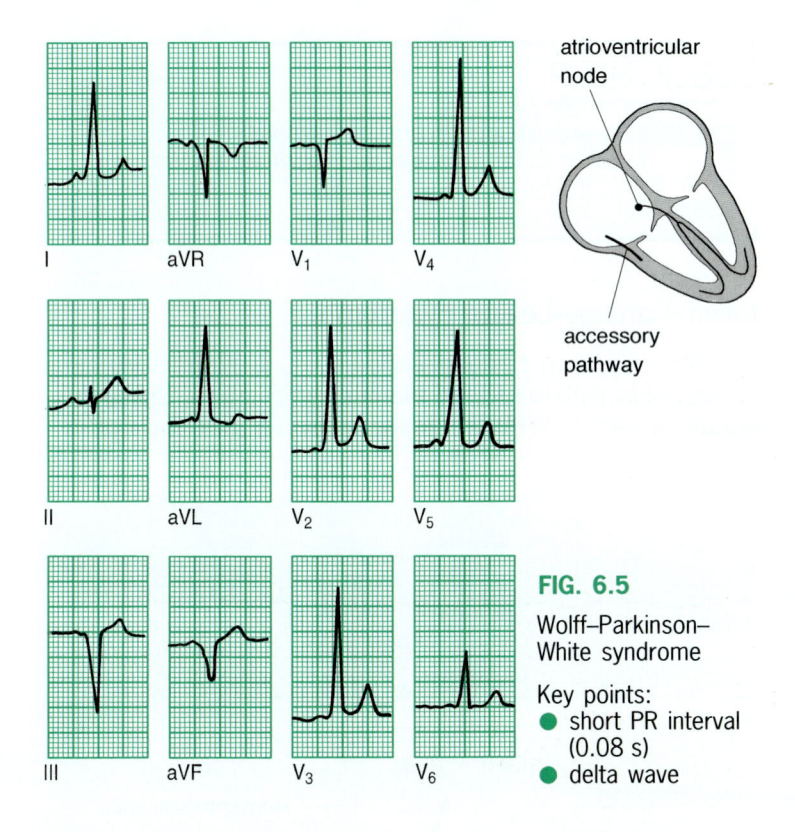

rise to a **delta wave** – the first part of the QRS complex (Fig. 6.4). Shortly afterwards, the rest of the ventricular muscle is depolarized rapidly with the arrival of the normally conducted wave of depolarization via the AV node.

Figure 6.5 shows a 12-lead ECG recorded from a patient with WPW syndrome.

WPW syndrome may be found incidentally and be asymptomatic – if so, no action is needed. Some patients develop palpitations due to an arrhythmia. The management of arrhythmias in WPW syndrome is discussed in detail on p. 48. If a patient with WPW syndrome requires surgery of any kind, the anaesthetist must be informed of the ECG findings.

114 MAKING SENSE OF THE ECG

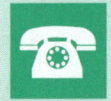

> **SEEK HELP**
>
> Referral to a cardiologist is appropriate if a patient with a short PR interval has experienced palpitations.

Lown–Ganong–Levine syndrome

Patients with Lown–Ganong–Levine (LGL) syndrome also have an accessory pathway (called the bundle of James). Unlike the bundle of Kent in WPW syndrome, however, the bundle of

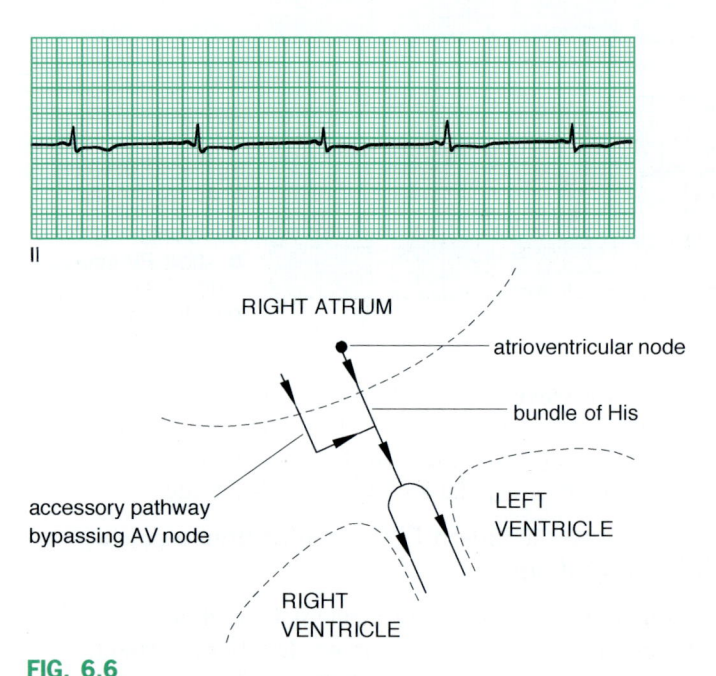

FIG. 6.6

Lown–Ganong–Levine syndrome

Key points: ● short PR interval (0.08 s)
● no delta wave

James does not activate the ventricular muscle directly. Instead, it simply connects the atria to the bundle of His (Fig. 6.6).

Because the accessory bundle allows the wave of depolarization to bypass the slowly conducting AV node, patients with LGL syndrome have a short PR interval. However, as there is no abnormal ventricular activation, there is no delta wave. LGL syndrome carries the same risk of paroxysmal tachycardias as WPW syndrome.

> ### SEEK HELP
> Referral to a cardiologist is appropriate if a patient with a short PR interval has experienced palpitations.

IS THE PR INTERVAL OVER 0.2 SECONDS LONG?

Prolongation of the PR interval is a common finding and indicates that conduction through the AV node has been delayed. When this delay is constant for each cardiac cycle, and each P wave is followed by a QRS complex, it is referred to as **first-degree AV block**.

First-degree AV block is normal when it accompanies a vagally induced bradycardia, as an increase in vagal tone decreases AV nodal conduction. It may also be a feature of:

- ischaemic heart disease
- hypokalaemia
- acute rheumatic myocarditis
- Lyme disease
- drugs
    - digoxin
    - quinidine
    - beta blockers
    - certain calcium-channel blockers.

FIG. 6.7

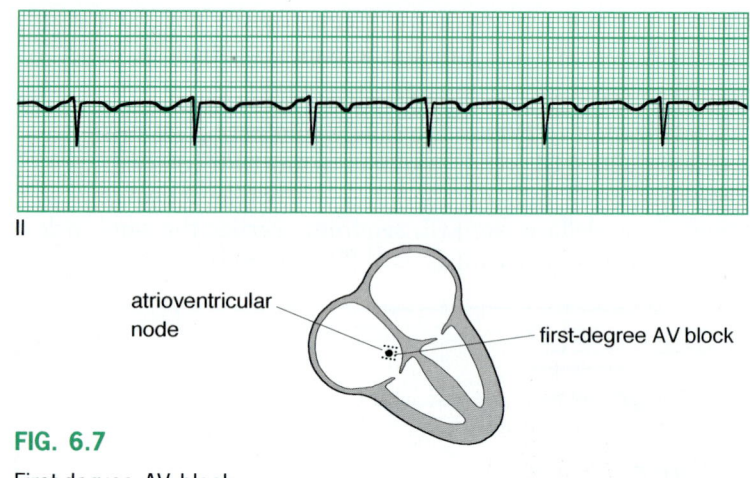

First-degree AV block

Key point: ● long PR interval (0.31 s)

Figure 6.7 shows a rhythm strip from a patient with first-degree AV block.

Look for a cause by taking a thorough patient history and, in particular, asking about any drug treatment the patient is currently receiving.

First-degree AV block in itself is asymptomatic and, in general, does not progress to other sorts of heart block (described later). No specific treatment is necessary for first degree AV block *in its own right,* but it should alert you to one of the above diagnoses (which may require treatment). It is **not** an indication for a pacemaker.

DOES THE PR INTERVAL VARY OR CAN IT NOT BE MEASURED?

Normally, the PR interval is constant. In some conditions, however, the interval between P waves and QRS complexes changes, giving rise to a variable PR interval. Sometimes a P wave is not followed by a QRS complex at all and so the PR interval cannot be measured.

If either, or both, of these occur, they indicate one of a number of possible AV conduction problems. These are distinguished by the relationship between P waves and QRS complexes:

- If the PR interval gradually lengthens with each beat, until one P wave fails to produce a QRS complex, the patient has **Mobitz type I AV block**.
- If the PR interval is fixed and normal, but occasionally a P wave fails to produce a QRS complex, the patient has **Mobitz type II AV block**.
- If alternate P waves are not followed by QRS complexes, the patient has **2:1 AV block**.
- If there is no relationship between P waves and QRS complexes, the patient has **third-degree (complete) AV block**.

All three types of AV block are discussed, with example ECGs, on the following pages. AV block was also discussed earlier in the book, on p. 60.

Mobitz type I AV block

Mobitz type I AV block is one of the types of second-degree heart block and is also known as the Wenckebach phenomenon. Its characteristic features are:

- The PR interval shows progressive lengthening until one P wave fails to be conducted and fails to produce a QRS complex.
- The PR interval resets to normal and the cycle repeats.

These features are demonstrated in the rhythm strip in Fig. 6.8.

Mobitz type I AV block is thought to result from abnormal conduction through the AV node itself and can result simply from periods of high vagal activity, so it sometimes occurs during sleep. It may also occur in generalized disease of the

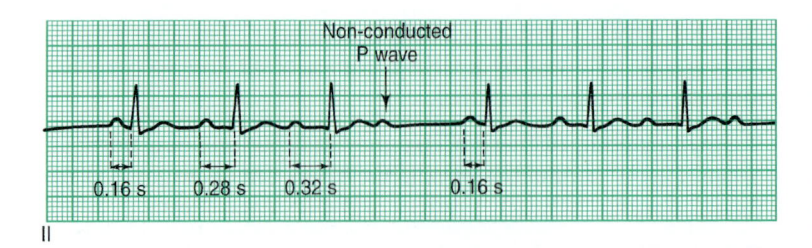

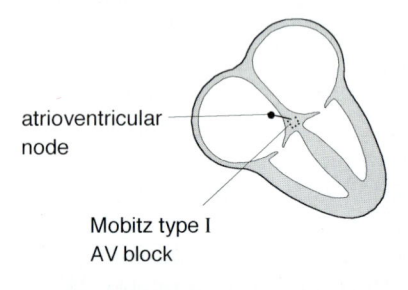

FIG. 6.8

Mobitz type I AV block

Key points:
- progressive lengthening of PR interval
- a P wave then fails to be conducted
- PR interval resets and cycle repeats

conducting tissues. It is regarded as a relatively benign form of AV block, and a permanent pacemaker is not required unless the frequency of 'dropped' ventricular beats causes a symptomatic bradycardia.

In acute myocardial infarction (MI), however, pacing may be required, depending upon the type of infarction. In **anterior** myocardial infarction, a prophylactic temporary pacemaker is recommended in case third-degree (complete) heart block develops. In **inferior** myocardial infarction, a pacemaker is only needed if symptoms or haemodynamic compromise results. Patients found to have Mobitz type I AV block prior to surgery will usually require temporary pacing perioperatively – discuss this with the anaesthetist and a cardiologist.

SEEK HELP

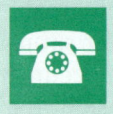

Mobitz type I AV block may require pacing. Seek the advice of a cardiologist without delay.

Mobitz type II AV block

Mobitz type II AV block is another type of second-degree heart block and its characteristic features are:

- Most P waves are followed by a QRS complex.
- The PR interval is normal and *constant*.
- Occasionally, a P wave is not followed by a QRS complex.

These features are demonstrated in the rhythm strip in Fig. 6.9.

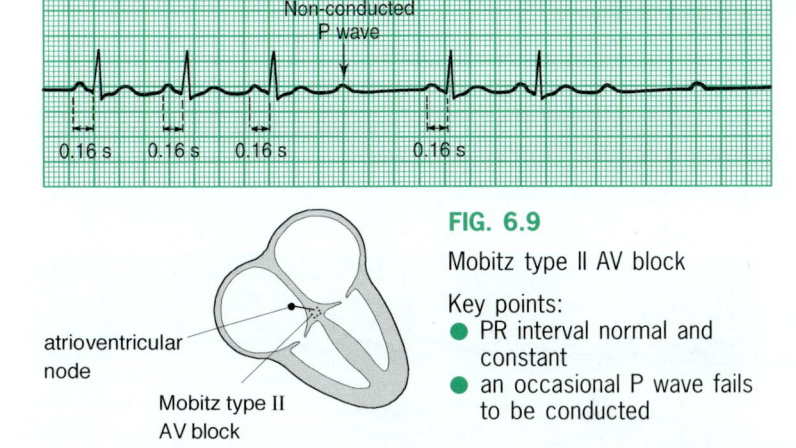

FIG. 6.9

Mobitz type II AV block

Key points:
- PR interval normal and constant
- an occasional P wave fails to be conducted

Mobitz type II AV block is thought to result from abnormal conduction below the AV node, in the bundle of His, and is considered more serious than Mobitz type I as it can progress without warning to third-degree (complete) heart block. Referral to a cardiologist is therefore recommended as a pacemaker may be required.

The indications for pacing Mobitz type II AV block in the setting of an acute MI, or perioperatively, are the same as for Mobitz type I AV block.

SEEK HELP

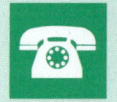

Mobitz type II AV block may require pacing. Seek the advice of a cardiologist without delay.

2:1 AV block

2:1 AV block is a special form of second-degree heart block in which alternate P waves are not followed by QRS complexes (Fig. 6.10).

2:1 AV block cannot be categorized as Mobitz type I or type II because it is impossible to say whether the PR interval for the non-conducted P waves would have been the same as, or longer than, the conducted P waves.

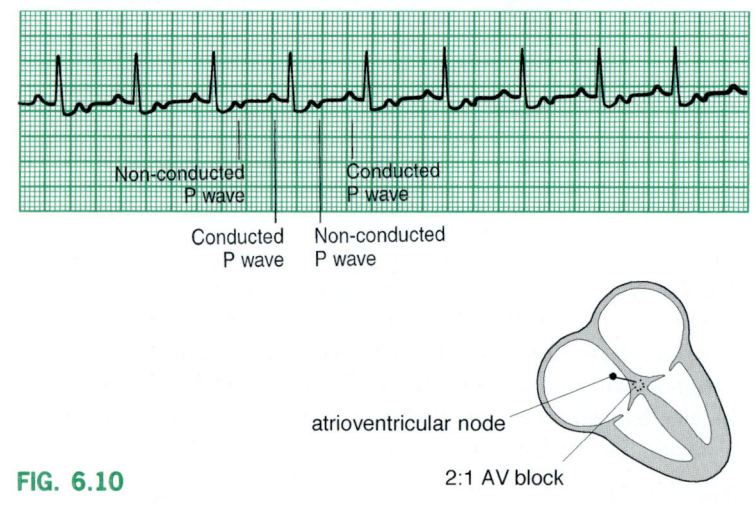

FIG. 6.10

2:1 AV block

Key point: ● alternate P waves fail to be conducted

Third-degree AV block

In third-degree AV block ('complete heart block'), there is complete interruption of conduction between atria and ventricles, so that the two are working independently. The atrial P waves bear no relationship to the ventricular QRS complexes, which usually arise as the result of a ventricular escape rhythm (p. 61). An example is shown in Fig. 6.11.

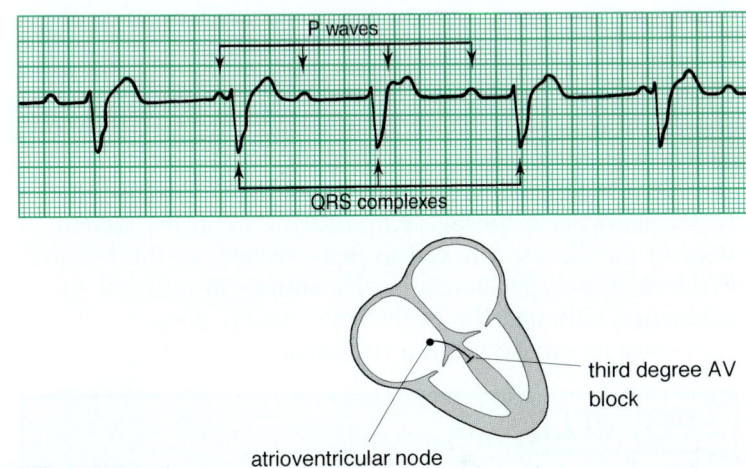

FIG. 6.11

Third-degree AV block

Key points:
- P wave (atrial) rate is 85 per minute
- QRS complex (ventricular) rate is 54 per minute
- broad QRS complexes
- no relationship between P waves and QRS complexes

It is important to remember that any atrial rhythm can coexist with third-degree heart block, and so the P waves may be abnormal or even absent. A combination of bradycardia (usually 15–40 beats per minute) and broad QRS complexes should alert you to suspect third-degree heart block.

In acute **inferior** wall myocardial infarction, third-degree AV block requires pacing if the patient is symptomatic or haemodynamically compromised. In acute **anterior** wall myocardial infarction, the development of third-degree AV block usually indicates an extensive infarct (and thus a poor prognosis). Temporary pacing is indicated regardless of the patient's symptoms or haemodynamic state. Temporary pacing is also usually necessary perioperatively in patients about to undergo surgery, who are found to have third-degree AV block.

In the elderly, third-degree AV block may cause heart failure, dizziness, falls or even loss of consciousness – permanent pacing is indicated under these circumstances.

Congenital varieties of third-degree AV block are uncommon and you should seek the advice of a cardiologist. In a young patient with a recent onset of third-degree AV block, always consider the possibility of Lyme disease. This is transmitted by the spirochaete *Borrelia burgdorferi* and, in the second stage of the illness, can lead to first-, second- or third-degree AV block. The AV block can resolve entirely in response to antibiotics, although the patient may require support with a temporary pacemaker during treatment.

SEEK HELP

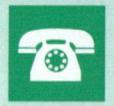

Third-degree AV block usually requires pacing. Seek the advice of a cardiologist without delay.

AV dissociation

AV dissociation is a term that is commonly used interchangeably with third-degree AV block; however, it does **not** mean the same thing. AV dissociation should only be used to describe the appearance of an escape rhythm (from the AV junction or ventricles) during sinus bradycardia. This can be distinguished from third-degree AV block by recognizing that the ventricular (QRS) rate is *higher* than the atrial (P wave) rate. The opposite is found in third-degree AV block.

Summary

To assess the PR interval, ask the following questions:

1. Is the PR interval less than 0.12 s long?

If 'yes', consider:
- Atrioventricular (AV) junctional rhythms
- Wolff–Parkinson–White syndrome
- Lown–Ganong–Levine syndrome

2. Is the PR interval over 0.2 s long?

If 'yes', consider:
- First-degree AV block
    - ischaemic heart disease
    - hypokalaemia
    - acute rheumatic myocarditis
    - Lyme disease
    - drugs
        - digoxin
        - quinidine
        - beta blockers
        - certain calcium-channel blockers

3. Does the PR interval vary or can it not be measured?

If 'yes', consider:
- Second-degree AV block
    - Mobitz type I (Wenckebach phenomenon)
    - Mobitz type II
    - 2:1 AV block
- Third-degree AV block

7

THE Q WAVE

After measuring the PR interval, go on to examine the QRS complex in each lead. Begin by looking for Q waves. A Q wave is present whenever the first deflection of the QRS complex points downwards (Fig. 7.1).

As you examine the QRS complex in each lead, the first question to ask is:

● Are there any 'pathological' Q waves?

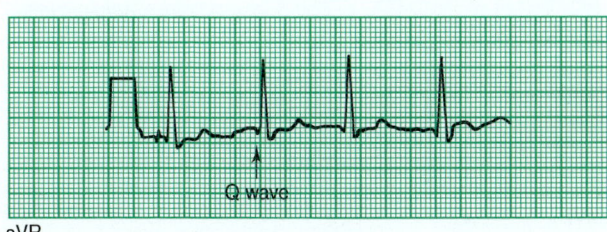

aVR

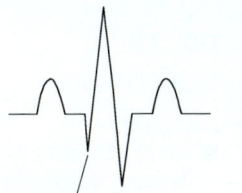

FIG. 7.1

The Q wave

Key point:
● Q wave is present when the first QRS deflection is downwards

Q wave

126 MAKING SENSE OF THE ECG

7

In this chapter we will help you to answer this question and to interpret any abnormality you may find.

ARE THERE ANY 'PATHOLOGICAL' Q WAVES?

If Q waves are present, begin by asking:

- Could these be normal?

Q waves are usually absent from *most* of the leads of a normal ECG. However, *small* Q waves are normal in leads that look at the heart from the left: I, II, aVL, V_5 and V_6.

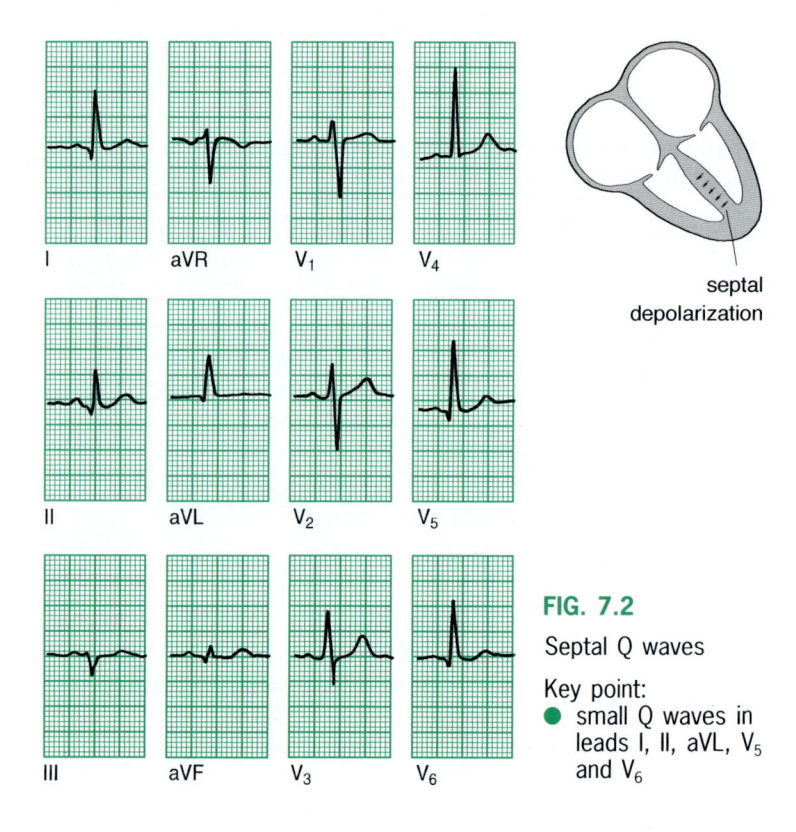

septal depolarization

FIG. 7.2

Septal Q waves

Key point:
- small Q waves in leads I, II, aVL, V_5 and V_6

THE Q WAVE

They result from septal depolarization, which normally occurs from left to right, and hence are referred to as 'septal' Q waves (Fig. 7.2).

A small Q wave may also be normal in lead III, and is often associated with an inverted T wave. Both may disappear on deep inspiration (Fig. 7.3).

Q waves in other leads are likely to be abnormal or **'pathological'**, particularly if they are:

- \> 2 small squares deep

or

- \> 25% of the height of the following R wave in depth

and/or

- \> 1 small square wide.

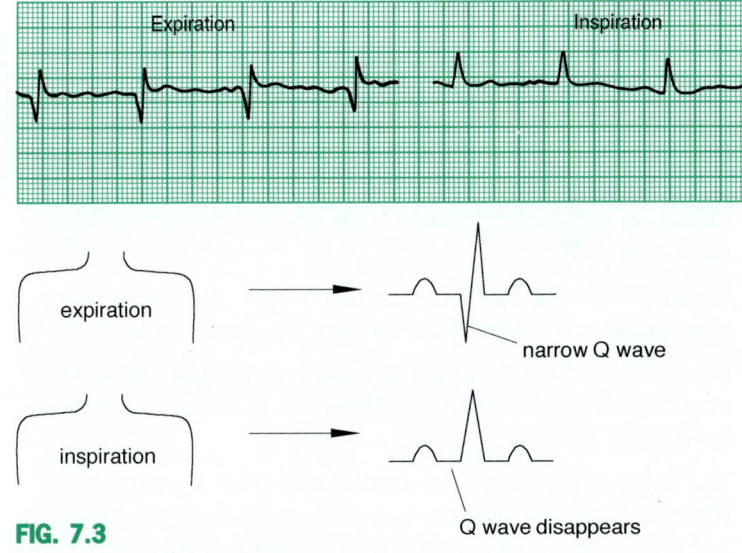

FIG. 7.3

Normal Q waves in lead III

Key points:
- narrow Q waves in lead III
- disappear on inspiration

If wide or deep Q waves (i.e. exceeding the above criteria) are present, consider:

- myocardial infarction
- left ventricular hypertrophy
- bundle branch block.

Myocardial infarction and left ventricular hypertrophy are discussed on the following pages. The bundle branch blocks are covered in detail in Chapter 8.

An abnormal Q wave (in lead III) is also a feature of:

- pulmonary embolism.

It is part of the 'classic' $S_I Q_{III} T_{III}$ pattern that is often quoted, although rarely seen. However, the Q_{III} rarely satisfies the 'pathological' Q wave criteria. The most frequent finding in pulmonary embolism is a tachycardia.

Myocardial infarction

Q waves start to appear within a few hours of the onset of myocardial infarction and in 90% of cases become permanent. The presence of Q waves alone therefore gives no clue as to the timing of the infarction. As with the other ECG changes in myocardial infarction, the location of the infarction can be determined from an analysis of the ECG leads (*see* Table 9.2).

Figure 7.4 shows an ECG recorded 5 days after an anterior myocardial infarction. Q waves have developed in leads V_1–V_4.

Figure 7.5 is from a patient who had an inferior myocardial infarction 2 years previously. Abnormal Q waves are seen in leads II, III and aVF.

The diagnosis of acute myocardial infarction is normally apparent from the presenting symptoms (chest pain, nausea and sweating) and ECG changes that are present (especially ST segment elevation), and can be confirmed by serial cardiac enzyme measurements. The management of acute myocardial infarction is discussed in detail on p. 156.

THE Q WAVE

FIG. 7.4

Anterior myocardial infarction (day 5)

Key points:
- Q waves in leads V_1–V_4
- T wave inversion in leads V_1–V_4

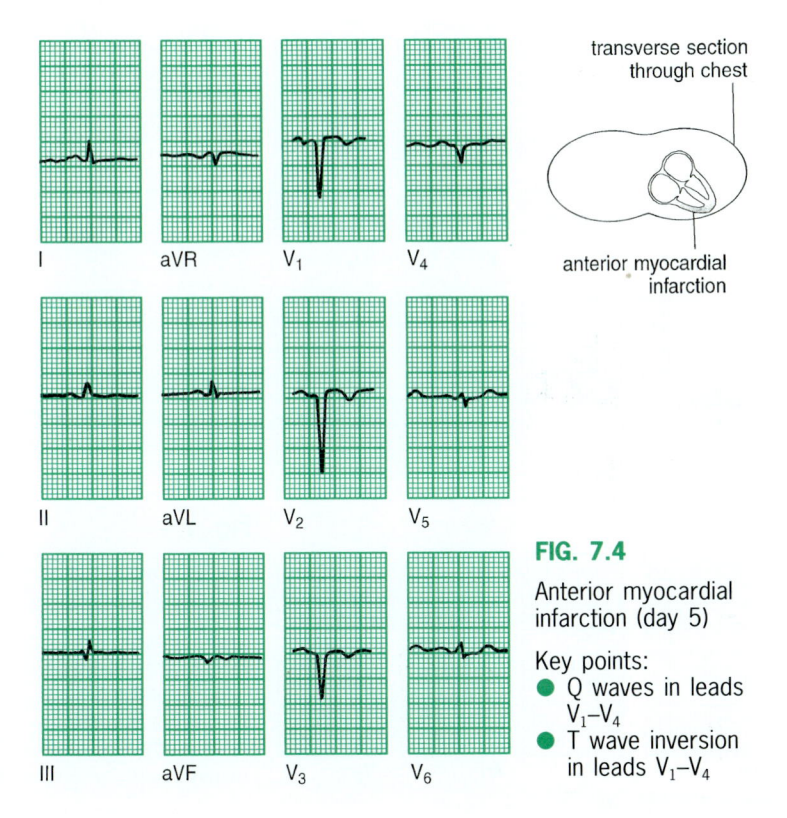

ACT QUICKLY

Acute myocardial infarction is a medical emergency. Prompt diagnosis and treatment are essential.

130 MAKING SENSE OF THE ECG

FIG. 7.5

Inferior myocardial infarction (year 2)

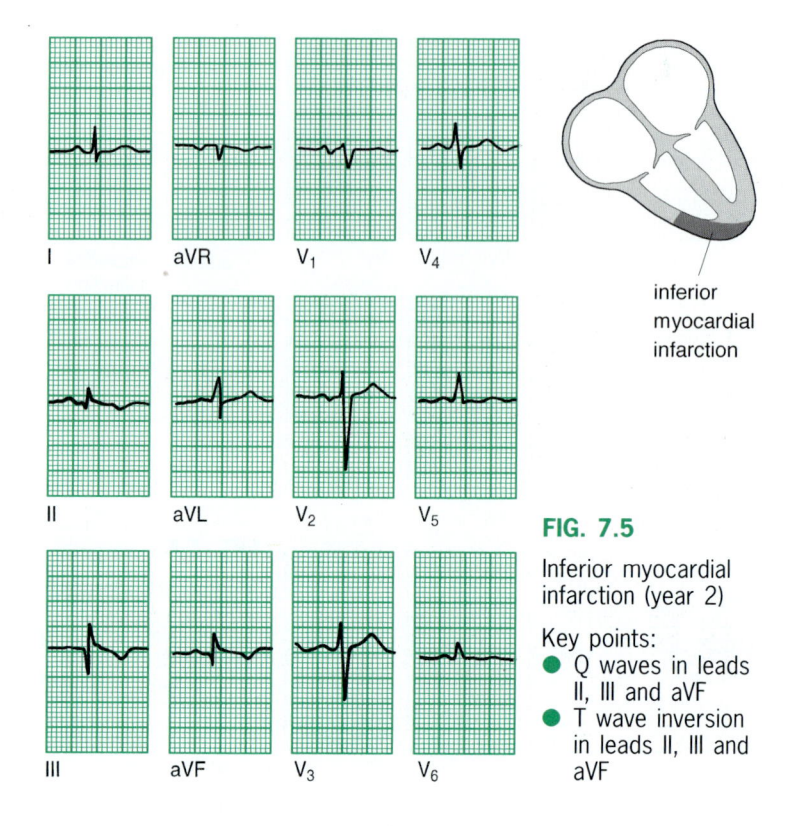

Key points:
- Q waves in leads II, III and aVF
- T wave inversion in leads II, III and aVF

When Q waves are found 'incidentally' on an ECG recorded for other reasons, a thorough review of the patient's history is necessary. Ask about:

- previous documented myocardial infarctions
- previous symptoms suggestive of myocardial infarction
- symptoms of recent myocardial ischaemia.

However, bear in mind that approximately 20% of myocardial infarctions are painless or 'silent'. If you remain uncertain about the significance of abnormal Q waves, and are suspicious about a previous myocardial infarction, there are a number of investigations that can help:

- **exercise ECG** (Chapter 15)
- **exercise thallium scintigraphy**
- **coronary angiography**.

A cardiologist will be able to advise you on which of these tests, if any, are appropriate.

Why do Q waves appear in myocardial infarction?

Q waves develop in myocardial infarction following the necrosis (or death) of an area of myocardium. The leads over the necrosed region can no longer record electrical activity in that area, and so they look 'through' it to record ventricular depolarization from 'within' the ventricular cavity rather than from outside.

Because each wave of depolarization flows from the inner surface of the heart to the outer, a lead recording the depolarization from a viewpoint 'within' the ventricle would 'see' the electrical activity flowing away from it; hence, the negative deflection on the ECG – the Q wave.

Left ventricular hypertrophy

At the start of this chapter, we said that small ('septal') Q waves can be a normal finding and result from depolarization of the interventricular septum. If the septum hypertrophies, its muscle mass (and hence the amount of electricity generated by depolarization) increases, and the Q waves become deeper.

Left ventricular hypertrophy often involves the septum, and so deep Q waves are often seen in leads looking at the left and inferior surfaces of the heart (Fig. 7.6).

Left ventricular hypertrophy is discussed more fully on p. 135.

FIG. 7.6

Left ventricular hypertrophy

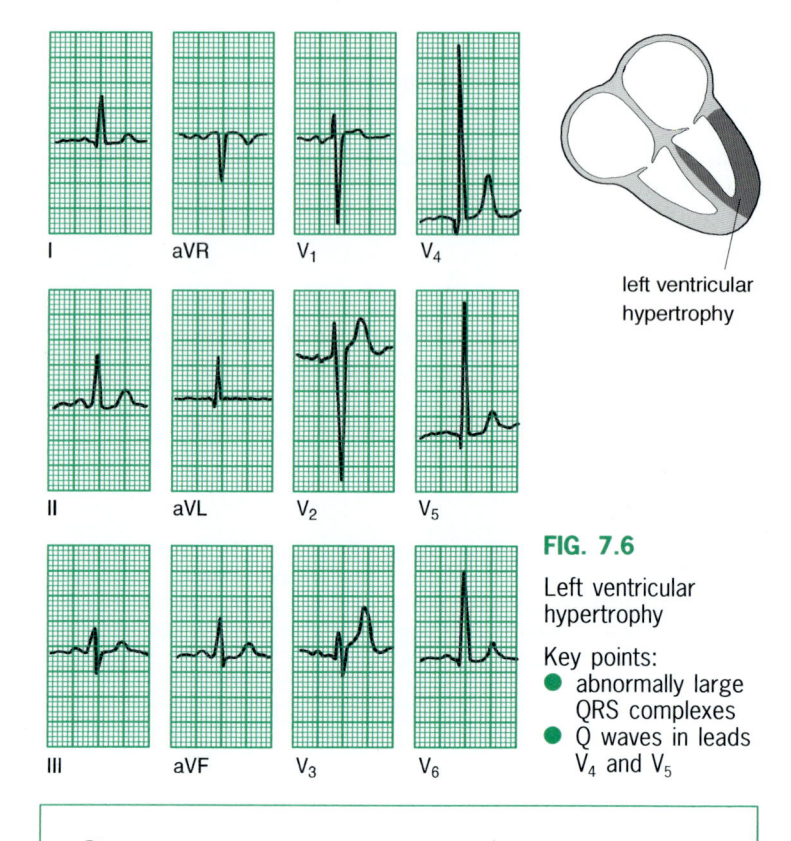

Key points:
- abnormally large QRS complexes
- Q waves in leads V_4 and V_5

Summary

To assess the Q wave, ask the following question:

1. Are there any 'pathological' Q waves?

If 'yes', consider:
- Myocardial infarction
- Left ventricular hypertrophy
- Bundle branch block

Also:
- Pulmonary embolism (although rarely 'pathological')

8

THE QRS COMPLEX

Normal QRS complexes have a different appearance in each of the 12 ECG leads (Fig. 8.1).

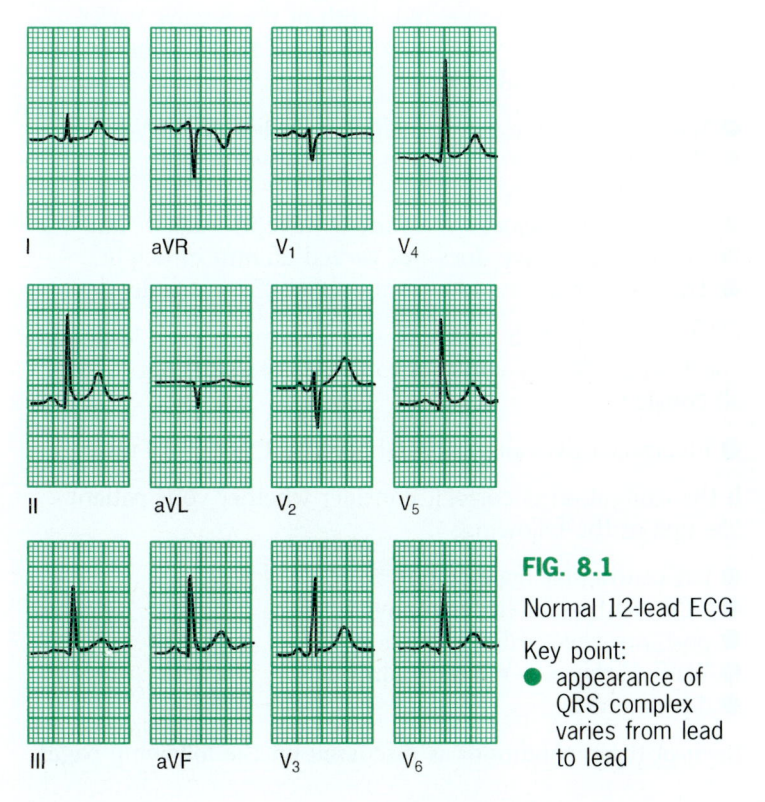

FIG. 8.1

Normal 12-lead ECG

Key point:
- appearance of QRS complex varies from lead to lead

When reviewing an ECG, look carefully at the size and shape of the QRS complexes in each lead and ask yourself the following four questions:

- Are any R or S waves too big?
- Are the QRS complexes too small?
- Are any QRS complexes too wide?
- Are any QRS complexes an abnormal shape?

In this chapter, we will help you to answer these questions and to interpret any abnormalities you may find.

ARE ANY R OR S WAVES TOO BIG?

The height of the R wave and depth of the S wave varies from lead to lead in the normal ECG (as Fig. 8.1 shows). As a rule, in the normal ECG:

- The R wave *increases* in height from lead V_1 to V_6.
- The R wave is *smaller* than the S wave in leads V_1 and V_2.
- The R wave is *bigger* than the S wave in leads V_5 and V_6.
- The tallest R wave does not exceed 25 mm in height.
- The deepest S wave does not exceed 25 mm in depth.

Always look carefully at the R and S waves in each lead, and check whether they conform to these criteria. If not, first of all consider:

- incorrect ECG calibration (should be 1 mV = 10 mm).

If the calibration is correct, consider whether your patient has one of the following:

- left ventricular hypertrophy
- right ventricular hypertrophy
- posterior myocardial infarction
- Wolff–Parkinson–White syndrome
- dextrocardia.

Each of these conditions is discussed on the following pages.

If the QRS complex is also abnormally wide, think of:

- bundle branch block

which is discussed later in this chapter.

Left ventricular hypertrophy

Hypertrophy of the left ventricle causes tall R waves in the leads that 'look at' the left ventricle – namely, I, aVL, V_5 and V_6 – and the reciprocal ('mirror image') change of deep S waves in leads that 'look at' the right ventricle – V_1 and V_2.

Left ventricular hypertrophy (LVH) should be suspected if *any* of the following criteria are met:

- The R wave in V_5 or V_6 exceeds 25 mm.
- The S wave in V_1 or V_2 exceeds 25 mm.
- The total of the R wave in V_5 or V_6 plus the S wave in V_1 or V_2 exceeds 35 mm.

These criteria are not diagnostic of LVH as young, thin people with normal hearts often have R and S waves outside these limits.

Figure 8.2 shows the ECG of a patient with LVH.

If evidence of LVH is present on the ECG, look too for evidence of 'strain':

- ST segment depression
- T wave inversion.

See Fig. 9.15 for an example of LVH with 'strain'.

Echocardiography is diagnostic for LVH. The treatment is usually that of the cause (Table 8.1).

Table 8.1 Causes of left ventricular hypertrophy

- Hypertension
- Aortic stenosis
- Coarctation of the aorta
- Hypertrophic cardiomyopathy

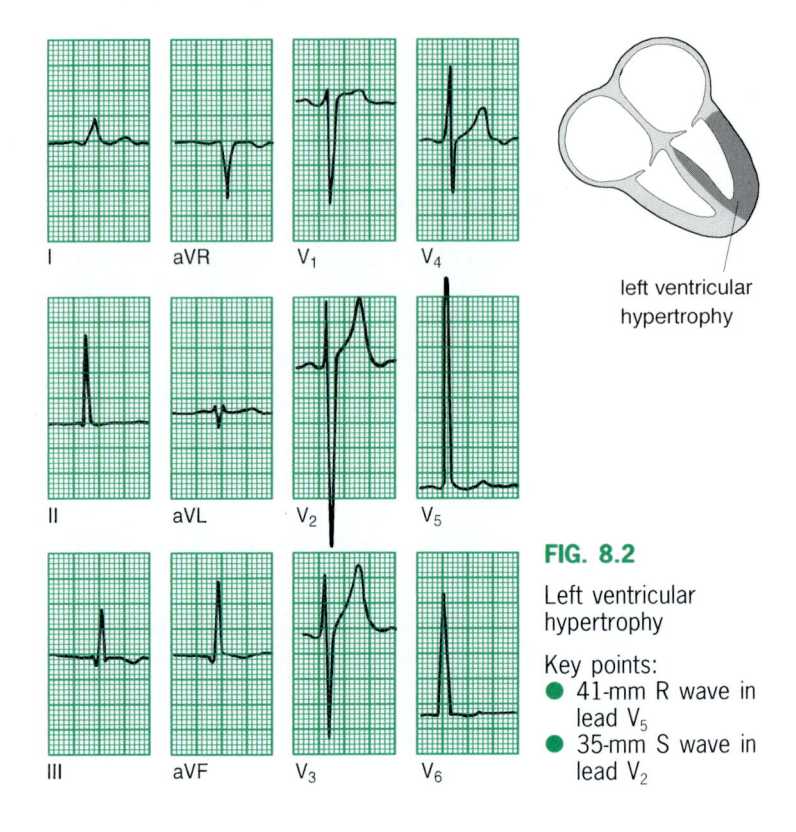

FIG. 8.2

Left ventricular hypertrophy

Key points:
- 41-mm R wave in lead V_5
- 35-mm S wave in lead V_2

Right ventricular hypertrophy

Right ventricular hypertrophy (RVH) causes a 'dominant' R wave (i.e. bigger than the S wave) in the leads that 'look at' the right ventricle, particularly V_1. RVH is also associated with:

- right axis deviation (Chapter 4)
- deep S waves in leads V_5 and V_6
- right bundle branch block

and, if 'strain' is present:

- ST segment depression
- T wave inversion.

THE QRS COMPLEX 137

FIG. 8.3

Right ventricular hypertrophy with 'strain'

Key points:
- dominant R waves in leads V_1–V_4
- deep S waves in leads V_5 and V_6
- right axis deviation
- ST segment depression/T wave inversion in leads V_1–V_3

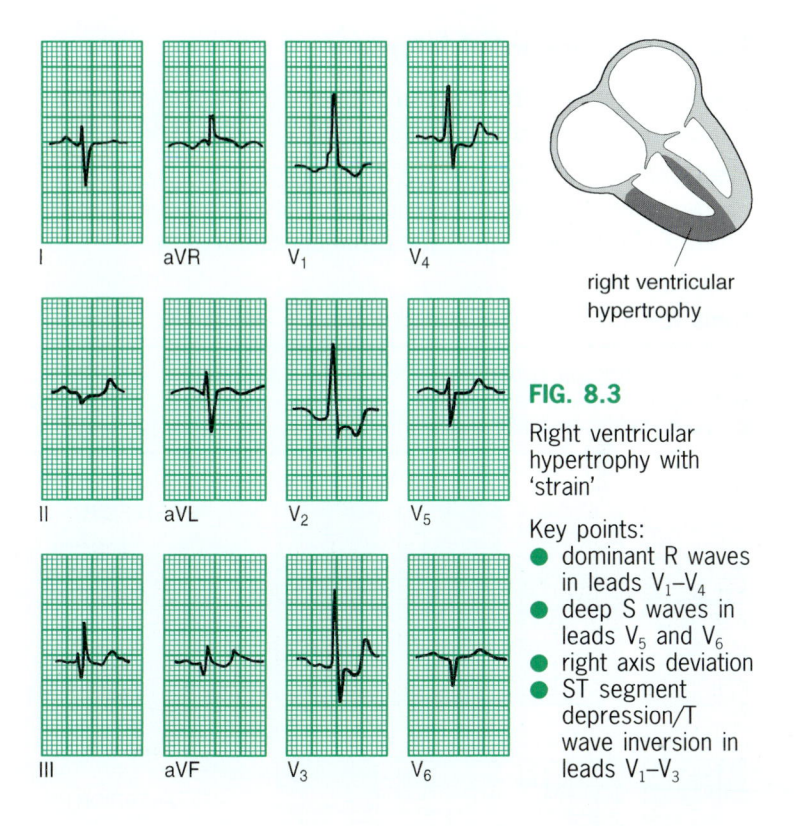

Figure 8.3 shows the ECG of a patient with RVH and 'strain'.

If you suspect RVH, look for an underlying cause (Table 8.2). The treatment of RVH is that of the underlying cause.

Table 8.2 Causes of right ventricular hypertrophy

- Pulmonary hypertension
- Pulmonary stenosis

Posterior myocardial infarction

Posterior myocardial infarction is one of a small number of causes of a 'dominant' R wave in lead V_1 (Table 8.3).

Infarction of the posterior wall of the left ventricle leads to reciprocal changes when viewed from the perspective of the anterior chest leads. Thus, the usual appearances of

Table 8.3 Causes of a 'dominant' R wave in lead V_1

- Right ventricular hypertrophy
- Posterior myocardial infarction
- Wolff–Parkinson–White syndrome (left-sided accessory pathway)

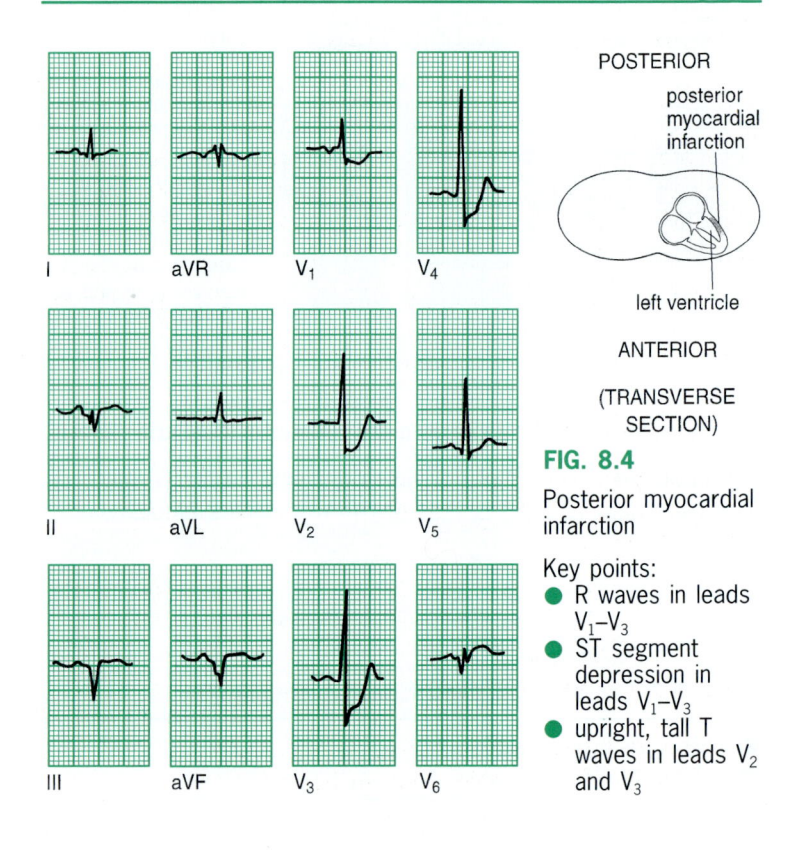

FIG. 8.4

Posterior myocardial infarction

Key points:
- R waves in leads V_1–V_3
- ST segment depression in leads V_1–V_3
- upright, tall T waves in leads V_2 and V_3

pathological Q waves, ST segment elevation and inverted T waves will appear as *R waves*, ST segment *depression* and *upright, tall* T waves when viewed from leads V_1–V_3 (Fig. 8.4).

The management of acute myocardial infarction is discussed in detail on p. 156.

> **ACT QUICKLY**
>
> Acute myocardial infarction is a medical emergency. Prompt diagnosis and treatment are essential.

Wolff–Parkinson–White syndrome

If you see a dominant R wave in leads V_1–V_3 in the presence of a short PR interval, think of Wolff–Parkinson–White (WPW) syndrome (p. 111). Patients with WPW syndrome have an accessory pathway (the bundle of Kent) that bypasses the AV node and bundle of His to connect the atria directly to the ventricles.

Accurate localization of the position of the accessory pathway can only be made with electrophysiological studies. Generally, however, a dominant R wave in leads V_1–V_3 indicates a left-sided accessory pathway, while a dominant S wave in leads V_1–V_3 indicates a right-sided accessory pathway.

The management of WPW syndrome is discussed in Chapter 6.

Dextrocardia

In dextrocardia, the heart lies on the right side of the chest instead of the left. The ECG does not show the normal progressive increase in R wave height across the chest leads; instead, the QRS complexes *decrease* in height across them (Fig. 8.5). In addition, the P wave is inverted in lead I and there is right axis deviation. **Right-sided chest leads** will show the pattern normally seen on the left.

140 MAKING SENSE OF THE ECG

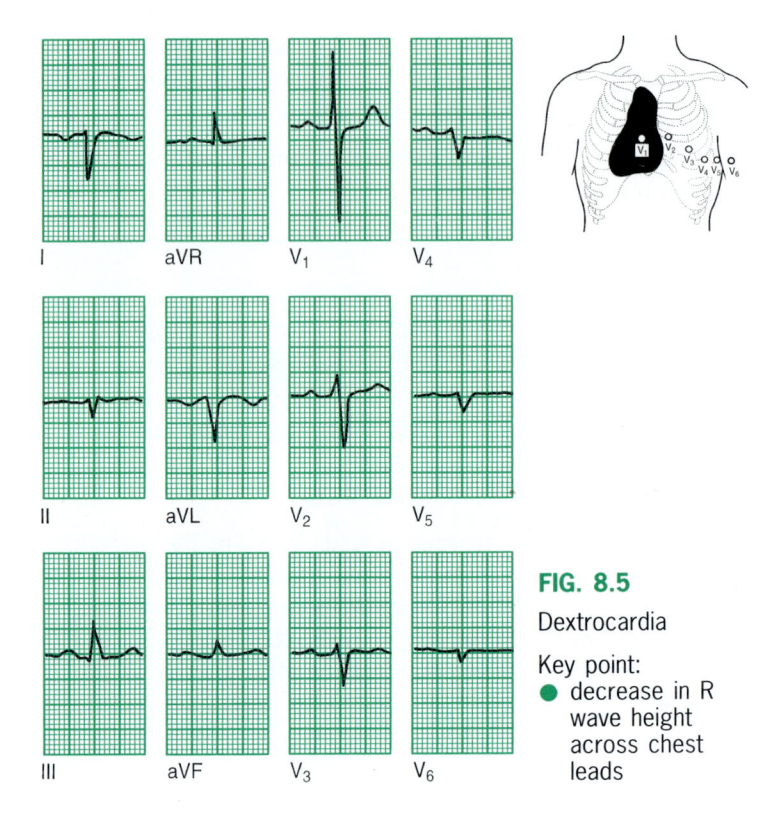

FIG. 8.5

Dextrocardia

Key point:
- decrease in R wave height across chest leads

If you suspect dextrocardia, check the location of the patient's apex beat. A chest X-ray is diagnostic. No specific treatment is required for dextrocardia, but ensure the condition is highlighted in the patient's notes and check for any associated syndromes (e.g. Kartagener's syndrome – dextrocardia, bronchiectasis and sinusitis).

ARE THE QRS COMPLEXES TOO SMALL?

Small QRS complexes indicate that relatively little of the voltage generated by ventricular depolarization is reaching the ECG electrodes. Although criteria exist for the normal upper limit of QRS complex size, there are no similar guidelines for the lower limit of QRS size.

Small QRS complexes may simply reflect a variant of normal. However, always check for:

- incorrect ECG calibration (should be 1 mV = 10 mm)

and also check whether the patient has:

- obesity
- emphysema.

Both of these conditions increase the distance between the heart and the chest electrodes.

However, if the QRS complexes appear small, and particularly if they have changed in relation to earlier ECG recordings, always consider the possibility of:

- pericardial effusion.

This is discussed on the following pages.

Pericardial effusion

A pericardial effusion reduces the voltage of the QRS complexes (Fig. 8.6).

Pericardial effusion can also cause electrical alternans, in which the height of the R waves and/or T waves alternates from beat to beat (Fig. 8.7).

A pericardial effusion may be asymptomatic when small. Larger effusions cause breathlessness and, ultimately, cardiac tamponade. The signs of Beck's triad indicate significant cardiac compromise:

- low blood pressure
- elevated jugular venous pressure
- impalpable apex beat.

In addition, the heart sounds are soft and there may be pulsus paradoxus (a marked fall in blood pressure on

142 MAKING SENSE OF THE ECG

FIG. 8.6

Pericardial effusion

Key point:
- small QRS complexes

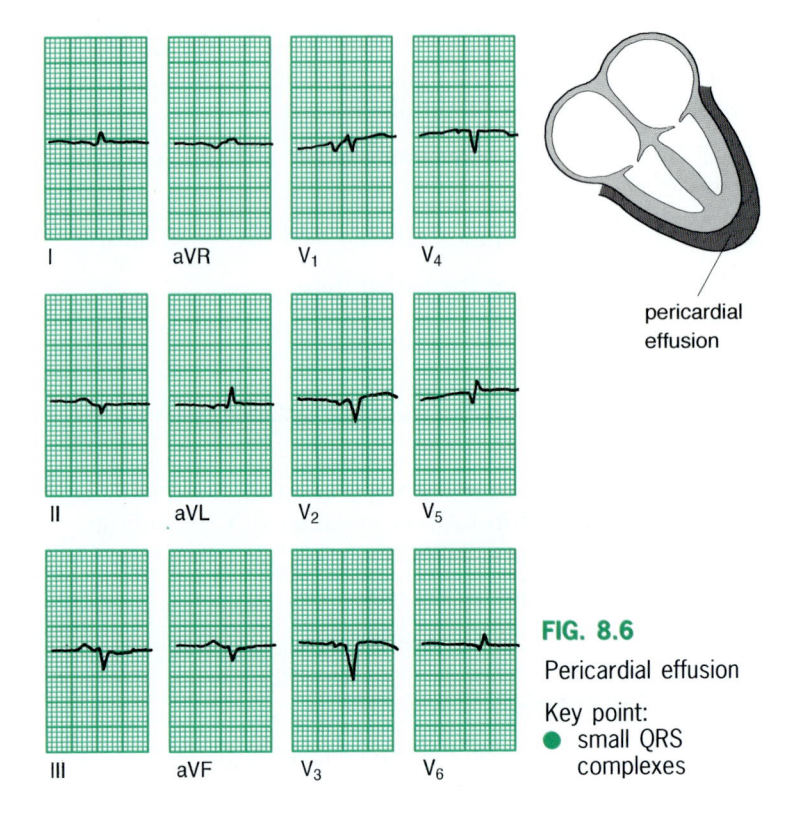

inspiration). The combination of small QRS complexes, electrical alternans and a tachycardia is a highly specific, but insensitive, indicator of a pericardial tamponade.

In a patient with a pericardial effusion, the chest X-ray may show a large globular heart but with no distension of the pulmonary veins. The echocardiogram is diagnostic.

Obtain the advice of a cardiologist immediately, particularly if the effusion is causing haemodynamic impairment. Urgent pericardial aspiration is required if the signs of tamponade are present, but should only be undertaken by, or under the guidance of, someone experienced in the procedure.

THE QRS COMPLEX

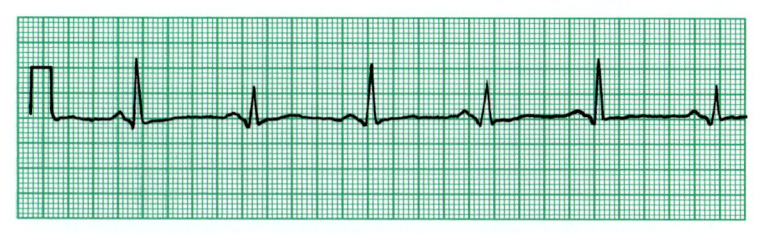

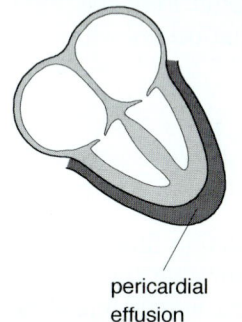

FIG. 8.7

Electrical alternans in pericardial effusion

Key point:
- variation in beat-to-beat R wave height

pericardial effusion

ACT QUICKLY

Cardiac tamponade is a medical emergency. Prompt diagnosis and treatment are essential.

ARE ANY QRS COMPLEXES TOO WIDE?

The QRS complex corresponds to depolarization of the ventricles, and this normally takes no longer than 0.12 s from start to finish. Thus, the width of a normal QRS complex is no greater than 3 small squares on the ECG.

Widening of the QRS complex is seen if conduction through the ventricles is slower than normal, and this usually means that depolarization has taken an abnormal route through the ventricles, as happens in:

- bundle branch block
- ventricular rhythms.

These conditions are discussed on the following pages.

Widening of the QRS complex can also result from the abnormal mechanism of depolarization that occurs with:

- hyperkalaemia.

Hyperkalaemia is discussed in detail on p. 181.

Bundle branch block

After leaving the bundle of His, the conduction fibres divide into two separate pathways as they pass through the interventricular septum – the left and right bundle branches – which supply the left and right ventricles respectively.

A block of either of the bundle branches delays the electrical activation of its ventricle, which must instead be depolarized *indirectly* via the other bundle branch. This prolongs the process of ventricular depolarization, and so the QRS complex is wider than 3 small squares. In addition, the shape of the QRS complex is distorted because of the abnormal pathway of depolarization.

In **left bundle branch block** (LBBB), the interventricular septum has to depolarize from right to left, a reversal of the normal pattern. This causes a small Q wave in lead V_1, and a small R wave in lead V_6 (Fig. 8.8). The right ventricle is depolarized normally via the right bundle branch, causing an R wave in lead V_1 and an S wave in lead V_6 (Fig. 8.9). Then, the left ventricle is depolarized by the right, causing an S wave in lead V_1 and another R wave (called R') in lead V_6 (Fig. 8.10).

Thus, the ECG of a patient with LBBB appears as in Fig. 8.11.

In **right bundle branch block** (RBBB), the interventricular septum depolarizes normally, from left to right, causing a

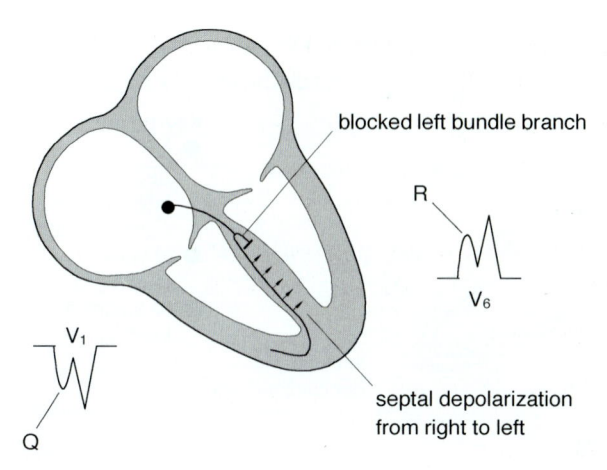

FIG. 8.8

Left bundle branch block

Key points:
- septal depolarization occurs from right to left
- small Q wave in lead V_1
- small R wave in lead V_6

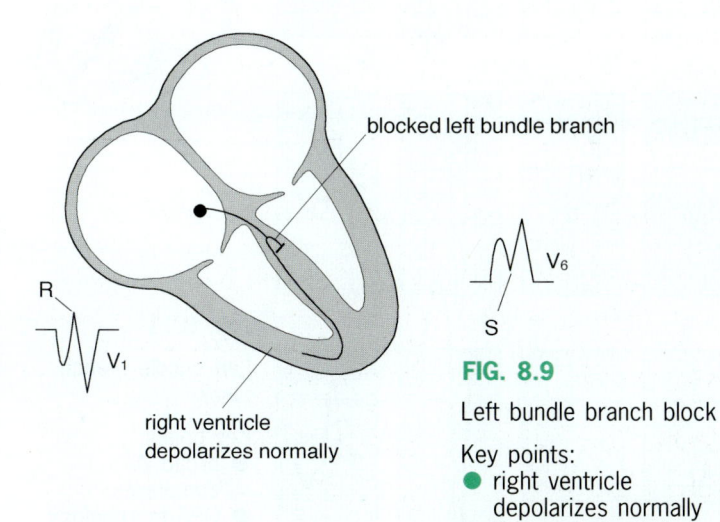

FIG. 8.9

Left bundle branch block

Key points:
- right ventricle depolarizes normally
- R wave in lead V_1
- S wave in lead V_6

FIG. 8.10

Left bundle branch block

Key points:
- left ventricle depolarizes late (by the right ventricle)
- S wave in lead V_1
- R' wave in lead V_6

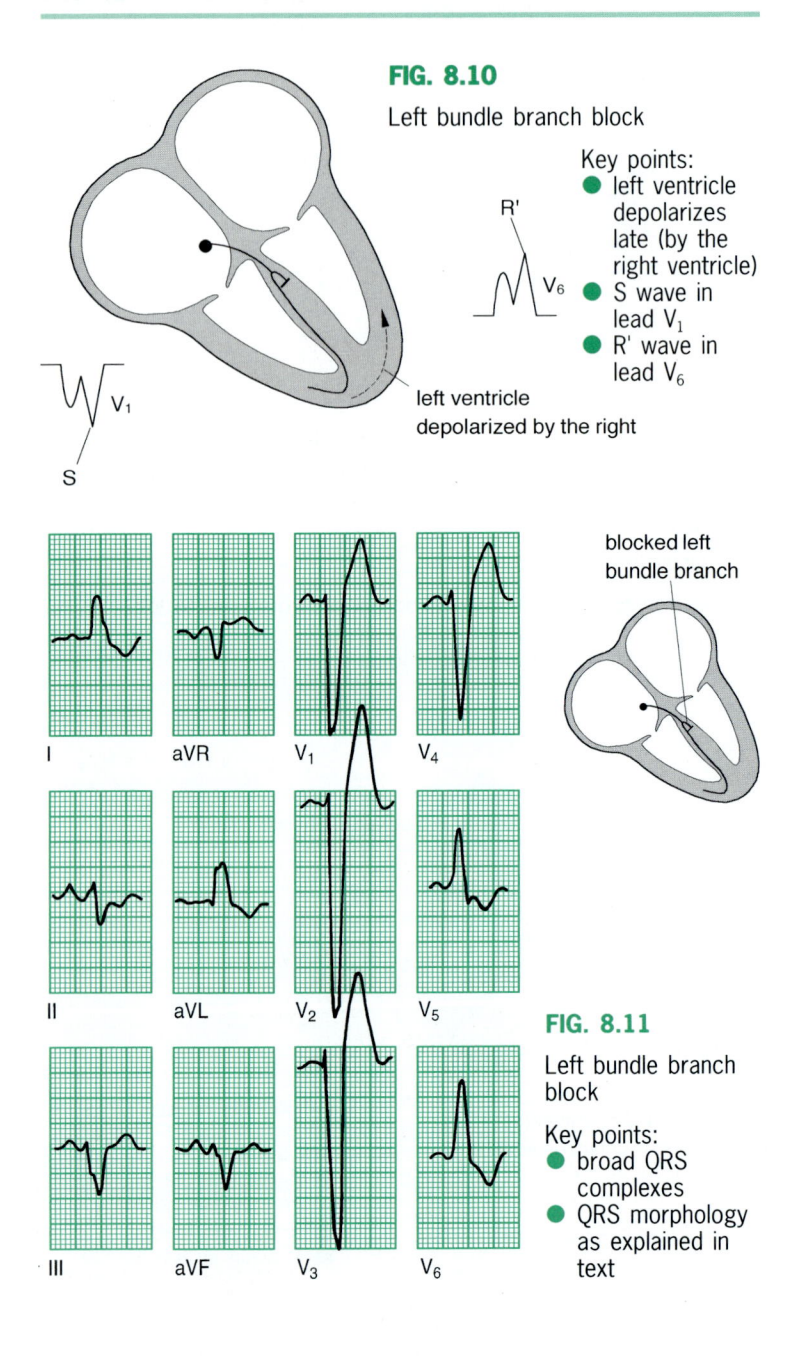

left ventricle depolarized by the right

blocked left bundle branch

FIG. 8.11

Left bundle branch block

Key points:
- broad QRS complexes
- QRS morphology as explained in text

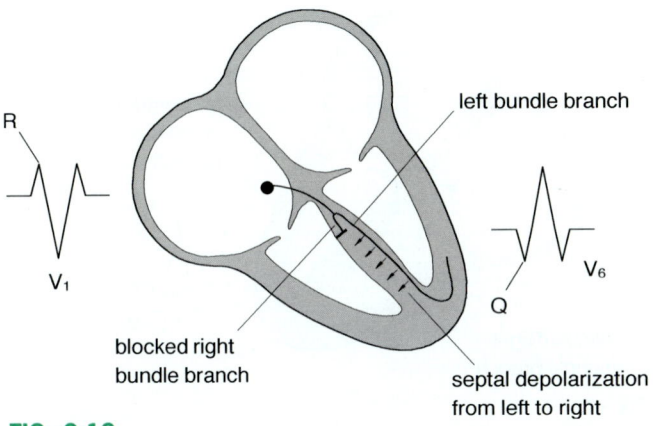

FIG. 8.12

Right bundle branch block

Key points:
- septum depolarization occurs from left to right
- small R wave in lead V_1
- small 'septal' Q wave in lead V_6

tiny R wave in lead V_1 and a small 'septal' Q wave in lead V_6 (Fig. 8.12). The left ventricle is depolarized normally via the left bundle branch, causing an S wave in lead V_1 and an R wave in lead V_6 (Fig. 8.13).

Then, the right ventricle is depolarized by the left, causing another R wave (called R') in lead V_1 and an S wave in lead V_6 (Fig. 8.14).

Thus, the ECG of a patient with RBBB appears as in Fig. 8.15.

An aide-memoire

Remembering the name 'William Morrow' should help you recall that:
- In left bundle branch block, the QRS looks like a 'W' in lead V_1 and an 'M' in lead V_6 (**William**')
- In right bundle branch block the QRS looks like an 'M' in lead V_1 and a 'W' in lead V_6 (**Morrow**')

148 MAKING SENSE OF THE ECG

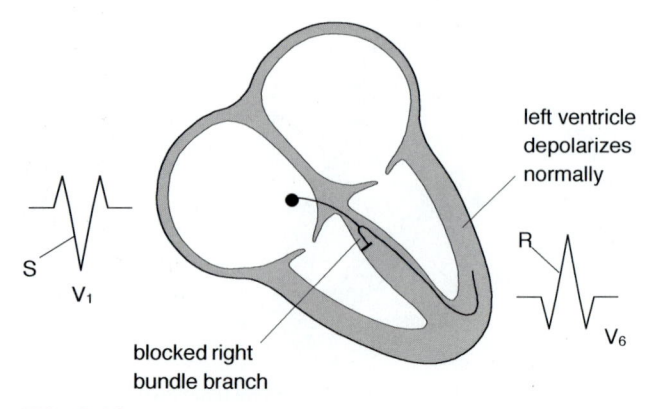

FIG. 8.13

Right bundle branch block

Key points:
- left ventricle depolarizes normally
- S wave in lead V_1
- R wave in lead V_6

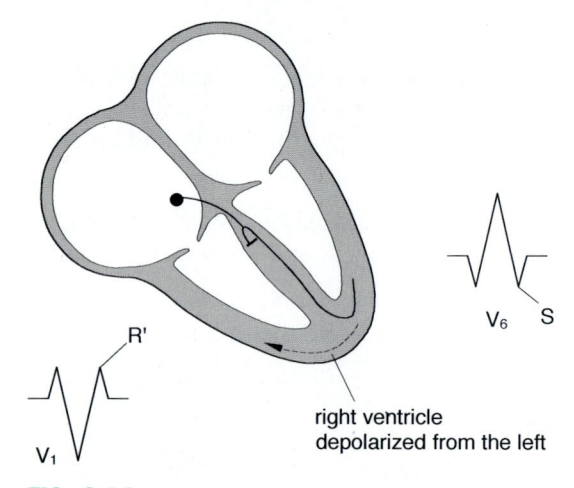

FIG. 8.14

Right bundle branch block

Key points:
- right ventricle depolarizes late (by the left ventricle)
- R' wave in lead V_1
- S wave in lead V_6

FIG. 8.15

Right bundle branch block

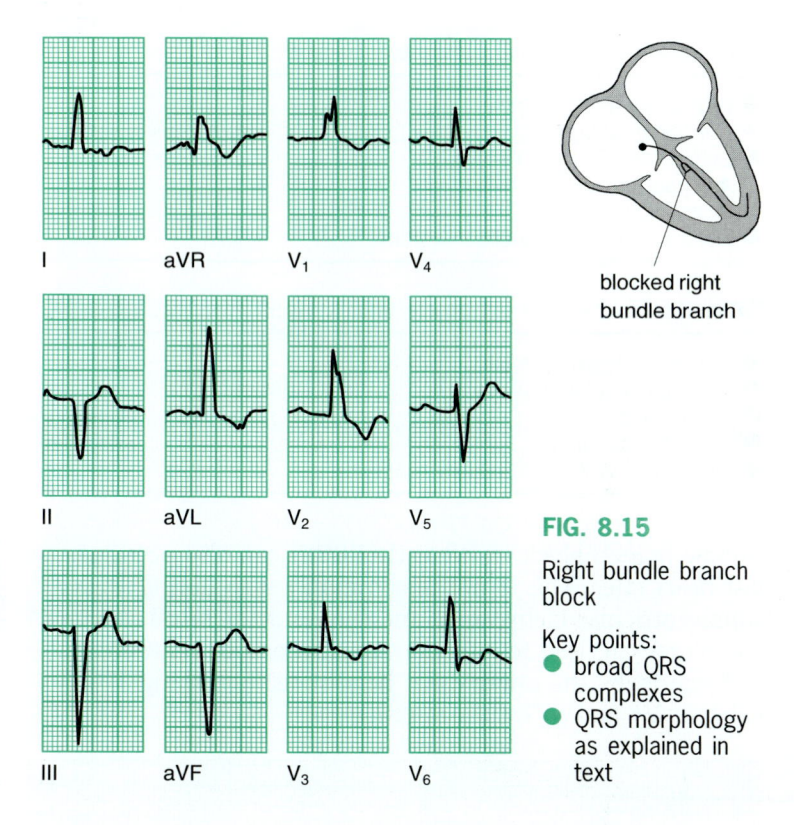

Key points:
- broad QRS complexes
- QRS morphology as explained in text

The presence of LBBB is almost invariably an indication of underlying pathology (Table 8.4), and the patient should be assessed accordingly. LBBB can be the presenting ECG feature of acute myocardial infarction, and is an indication for thrombolysis. The presence of LBBB renders interpretation of the ECG beyond the QRS complex impossible.

In contrast to LBBB, RBBB is a relatively common finding in otherwise normal hearts. However, it too can result from underlying disease (Table 8.5) and should be investigated according to the clinical presentation.

Table 8.4 Causes of left bundle branch block

- Ischaemic heart disease
- Cardiomyopathy
- Left ventricular hypertrophy
  - hypertension
  - aortic stenosis
- Fibrosis of the conduction system

Table 8.5 Causes of right bundle branch block

- Ischaemic heart disease
- Cardiomyopathy
- Atrial septal defect
- Ebstein's anomaly
- Pulmonary embolism (usually massive)

Bundle branch block (particularly RBBB) can also occur at fast heart rates. This is not uncommonly seen during supraventricular tachycardia, and the resultant broad complexes can lead to an incorrect diagnosis of ventricular tachycardia by the unwary. For help in distinguishing between VT and SVT, turn to p. 73.

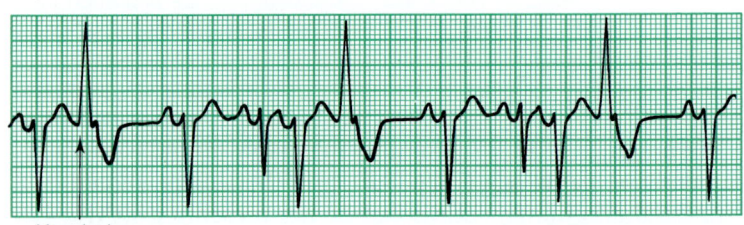

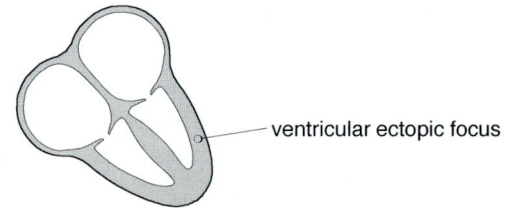

FIG. 8.16

Ventricular ectopic

Key points:
- broad QRS complex
- complex occurs earlier than expected

Both LBBB and RBBB are asymptomatic in themselves, and do not require treatment in their own right. Even so, they should prompt you to look for an underlying cause as appropriate to the patient's presentation.

Ventricular rhythms

When depolarization is initiated from within the ventricular muscle itself, the wave of electrical activity has to spread from myocyte to myocyte rather than using the more rapid Purkinje network. This prolongs the process of ventricular depolarization and thus widens the QRS complex (Fig. 8.16).

For more information about ventricular rhythms, and help with their identification, turn back to Chapter 3.

ARE ANY QRS COMPLEXES AN ABNORMAL SHAPE?

Most of the causes of an abnormally shaped QRS complex have already been discussed earlier in this chapter. However, occasionally you will encounter QRS complexes which just appear unusual without fitting any of these specific criteria.

You may see complexes which appear 'slurred', or have an abnormal 'notch', without necessarily being abnormally tall, small or wide. If this is the case, consider the following possible causes:

- incomplete bundle branch block
- fascicular block
- Wolff–Parkinson–White syndrome.

Further information on each of these can be found on the following pages.

Incomplete bundle branch block

Bundle branch block was discussed earlier in this chapter. Sometimes, however, conduction down a bundle branch can

Summary

To assess the QRS complex, ask the following questions:

1. Are any R or S waves too big?

If 'yes', consider:
- Incorrect ECG calibration
- Left ventricular hypertrophy
- Right ventricular hypertrophy
- Posterior myocardial infarction
- Wolff–Parkinson–White syndrome (left-sided accessory pathway)
- Dextrocardia

Also:
- Bundle branch block

2. Are the QRS complexes too small?

If 'yes', consider:
- Incorrect ECG calibration
- Obesity
- Emphysema
- Pericardial effusion

3. Are any QRS complexes too wide?

If 'yes', consider:
- Bundle branch block
- Ventricular rhythms

Also:
- Hyperkalaemia

4. Are any QRS complexes an abnormal shape?

If 'yes', consider:
- Incomplete bundle branch block
- Fascicular block
- Wolff–Parkinson–White syndrome

9

THE ST SEGMENT

The ST segment lies between the end of the S wave and the start of the T wave. Normally, the ST segment is isoelectric, meaning that it lies at the same level as the ECG's baseline, the horizontal line between the end of the T wave and the start of the P wave (Fig. 9.1).

ST segments can be abnormal in one of two ways, so the questions you need to ask about the ST segments when you review them are:

- Are the ST segments elevated?
- Are the ST segments depressed?

In this chapter, we will help you to answer these questions, and guide you on what to do next if you find an abnormality.

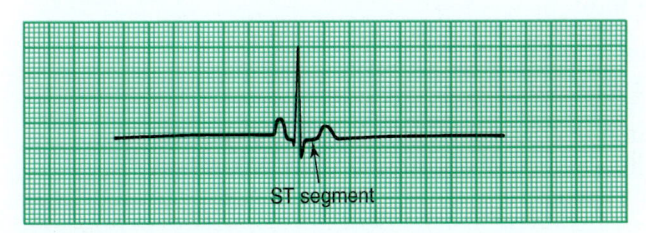

FIG. 9.1
The ST segment
Key point: • ST segment is normally isoelectric

ARE THE ST SEGMENTS ELEVATED?

Look carefully at the ST segment in each lead to see if it is isoelectric. If it is raised above this level, the ST segment is elevated.

ST segment elevation should never be ignored as it frequently indicates a serious problem that warrants urgent attention. If you see ST elevation in any lead, consider the following possible diagnoses:

- acute myocardial infarction
- left ventricular aneurysm
- Prinzmetal's (vasospastic) angina
- pericarditis
- high take-off.

Therefore, ST segment elevation can represent anything from a potentially life-threatening condition to a normal variant, making it particularly important to identify the cause. To help you in this task, we have described each of these five conditions (together with example ECGs) on the pages that follow.

Acute myocardial infarction

By definition, myocardial infarction causes permanent damage to the heart muscle. Myocardial infarction is often classified into:

- Q wave infarcts
- non-Q wave infarcts.

This section is chiefly concerned with Q wave infarction. Further information about **non-Q wave infarction** can be found in Chapter 10.

In **Q wave myocardial infarction**, the ECG changes gradually 'evolve' in the sequence shown in Fig. 9.2. The earliest change is ST segment elevation accompanied, or even preceded, by tall 'hyperacute' T waves. Over the next

THE ST SEGMENT

(1) Tall 'hyperacute' T waves

(2) ST segment elevation

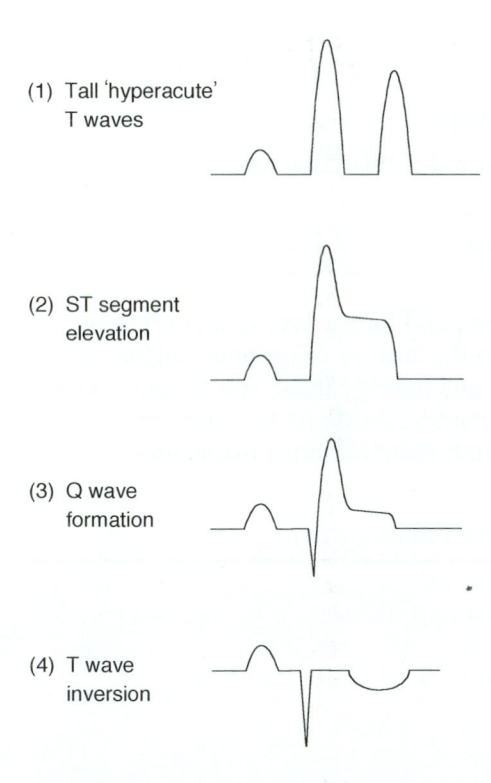

(3) Q wave formation

(4) T wave inversion

FIG. 9.2

Evolution of a Q wave myocardial infarction

few hours or days, Q waves appear, the ST segments return to normal and the T waves become inverted. It is usual for some permanent abnormality of the ECG to persist following myocardial infarction – usually 'pathological' Q waves, although the T waves may remain inverted permanently too.

Do not forget that acute myocardial infarction can also present with the new onset of **left bundle branch block** on the ECG (Chapter 8). Remember too that a **normal** ECG does not exclude an acute myocardial infarction.

Acute myocardial infarction requires urgent treatment and you must lose no time in trying to make the diagnosis. The diagnosis is established if at least two of the following three criteria are consistent with a myocardial infarction:

- patient's history
- ECG changes
- cardiac enzyme changes.

The symptoms of myocardial infarction are:

- tight, central chest pain
- nausea and vomiting
- sweating.

The pain is more severe, and longer lasting, than that of angina. Always ask about a history of previous angina or myocardial infarction, and assess cardiac risk factors (Table 9.1) and any possible contraindications to aspirin or thrombolysis. A thorough examination is mandatory.

Table 9.1 Risk factors for coronary artery disease

Modifiable:
- Cigarette smoking
- Hypertension
- Diabetes mellitus
- Hyperlipidaemia

Non-modifiable
- Age
- Male sex
- Family history

The cardiac enzymes (which are not *specifically* cardiac in origin) commonly measured in myocardial infarction are:

- creatine kinase (CK) or its isoenzyme, (CK-MB)
- aspartate transaminase (AST)
- lactate dehydrogenase (LDH).

The enzyme levels peak at different times after the onset of the infarction (Fig. 9.3).

You can see from Fig. 9.3 that significant changes in the cardiac enzymes may not be apparent for several hours after

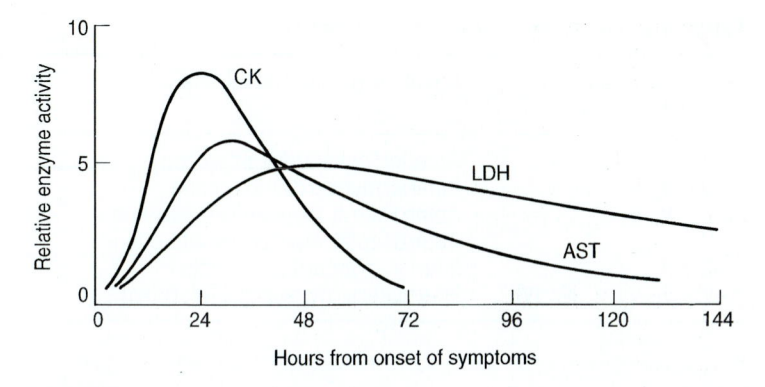

FIG. 9.3

Time course of enzyme levels after myocardial infarction

Key points:
- CK peaks after 24 h
- AST peaks after 30 h
- LDH peaks after 48 h

the onset of an infarction. Cardiac enzymes therefore have little role to play in the *initial* diagnosis of a myocardial infarction, and it is not at all unusual for enzyme levels to be normal upon admission.

Aortic dissection

Always beware of missing a diagnosis of aortic dissection. This too can cause ST segment elevation (if the dissection involves the coronary arteries) and chest pain, but patients may also complain of a 'tearing' back pain, have a different blood pressure in each arm and have mediastinal widening on their chest X-ray.

Having diagnosed myocardial infarction, waste no time in admitting the patient to a coronary care unit or other monitored area for treatment as indicated. This is discussed later in this section.

160 MAKING SENSE OF THE ECG

Table 9.2 Localization of myocardial infarctions

Leads containing ST segment elevation	Location of myocardial infarction
V_1–V_4	Anterior myocardial infarction
I, aVL, V_5–V_6	Lateral myocardial infarction
I, aVL, V_1–V_6	Anterolateral myocardial infarction
V_1–V_3	Anteroseptal myocardial infarction
II, III, aVF	Inferior myocardial infarction
I, aVL, V_5–V_6, II, III, aVF	Inferolateral myocardial infarction

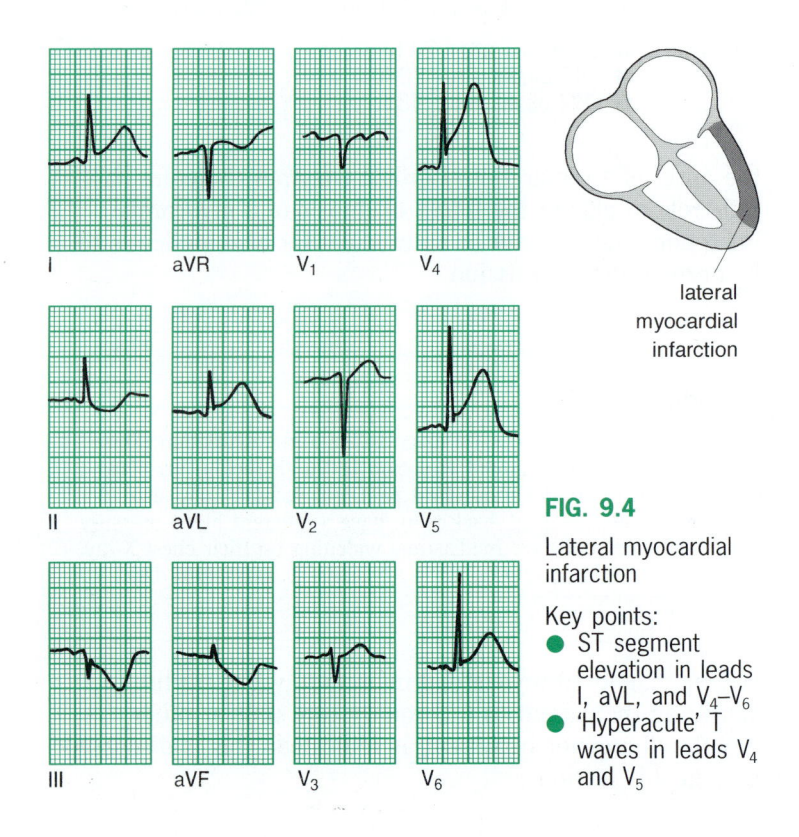

lateral myocardial infarction

FIG. 9.4

Lateral myocardial infarction

Key points:
- ST segment elevation in leads I, aVL, and V_4–V_6
- 'Hyperacute' T waves in leads V_4 and V_5

THE ST SEGMENT 161

The ECG also allows you to identify the area of myocardium damaged by the infarction, as the leads 'looking at' that area will be the ones in which abnormalities are seen (Table 9.2). Examples of myocardial infarctions affecting different areas are shown in Figs 9.4 – 9.6.

If you diagnose an inferior myocardial infarction, you must go on to ask the question:

● Is the right ventricle involved?

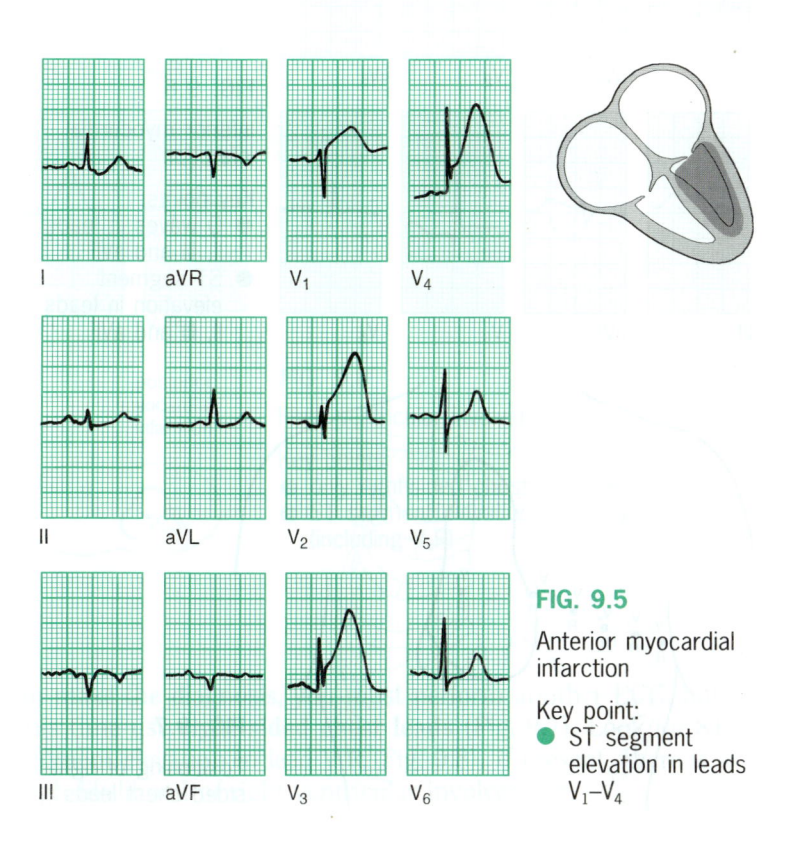

FIG. 9.5

Anterior myocardial infarction

Key point:
● ST segment elevation in leads V_1–V_4

> **Why is right ventricular infarction important?**
>
> Patients with a right ventricular infarction may develop the signs of right-sided heart failure (elevated jugular venous presure and peripheral oedema). The left ventricle may be functioning entirely normally, and the lungs are therefore clear. If these patients develop hypotension, it is usually because their left-sided filling pressure is too low (as the supply of blood from the damaged right ventricle is inadequate). Vasodilator drugs must be avoided, and intravenous fluids may be needed to maintain right ventricular output and thus ensure sufficient blood is supplied to the left ventricle. It may seem paradoxical to give intravenous fluids to patients who already appear to be in right heart failure, unless the reasons for doing so are understood. If haemodynamically compromised, these patients need monitoring of fluid balance using a Swan–Ganz catheter (to allow measurement of both right- and, indirectly, left-sided filling pressure). The risk of severe complications is high in these patients.

Patients with acute myocardial infarction require:

- pain relief (an opiate intravenously + antiemetic)
- oxygen
- aspirin, 150 mg orally.

Unless contraindicated, **thrombolysis** should be offered to all patients whose history suggests a myocardial infarction within the last 12 h and whose ECG shows:

- ST segment elevation consistent with infarction

or

- new left bundle branch block.

Following a myocardial infarction, patients should continue with:

- aspirin, 150 mg daily
- a beta blocker (e.g. timolol, 5 mg twice daily)
- an angiotensin-converting enzyme inhibitor if they exhibit signs of heart failure during the hospital stay.

THE ST SEGMENT 165

ACT QUICKLY

> Acute myocardial infarction is a medical emergency. Prompt diagnosis and treatment are essential.

Left ventricular aneurysm

The development of a left ventricular aneurysm is a late complication of myocardial infarction, seen (to varying degrees) in around 10% of survivors. The presence of an aneurysm can lead to persistent ST segment elevation in those chest leads that 'look at' the affected region (Fig. 9.9).

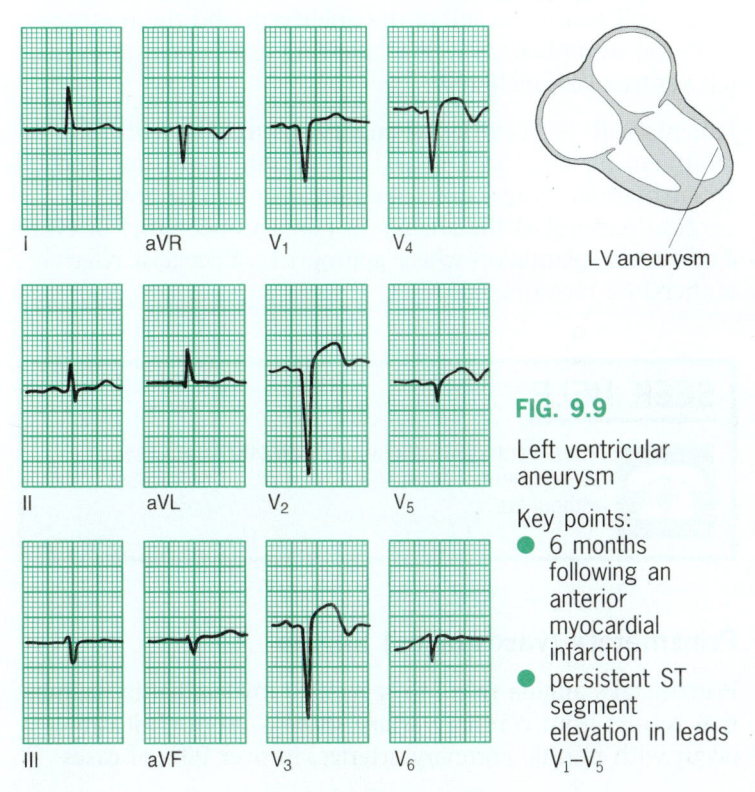

FIG. 9.9

Left ventricular aneurysm

Key points:
- 6 months following an anterior myocardial infarction
- persistent ST segment elevation in leads V_1–V_5

Ask the patient about a history of previous myocardial infarction, and assess the patient for symptoms and signs related to the aneurysm itself. Aneurysms, being non-contractile, can lead to left ventricular dysfunction and thrombus formation. They can also be a focus for arrhythmia formation. Presenting symptoms can therefore result from:

- heart failure
- embolic events
- arrhythmias.

The clinical signs of a left ventricular aneurysm are a 'double impulse' on precordial palpation and a fourth heart sound on auscultation. A chest X-ray may reveal a bulge on the cardiac outline. The investigation of choice is echocardiography which will reveal the site of the aneurysm and the presence of mural thrombus, as well as allowing assessment of overall left ventricular function.

Patients with left ventricular aneurysms may benefit from treatment for heart failure, and use of anticoagulation and antiarrhythmic drugs. Consideration may also be given to surgical removal of the aneurysm (aneurysmectomy) or even cardiac transplantation where appropriate. Specialist referral is therefore recommended.

SEEK HELP

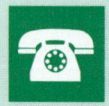

A left ventricular aneurysm warrants specialist assessment. Obtain the advice of a cardiologist without delay.

Prinzmetal's (vasospastic) angina

Prinzmetal's angina refers to reversible myocardial ischaemia that results from coronary artery spasm. Although it can occur with normal coronary arteries, in over 90% of cases

FIG. 9.10

Prinzmetal's (vasospastic) angina

Key point:
- anterior ST segment elevation during episode of chest pain

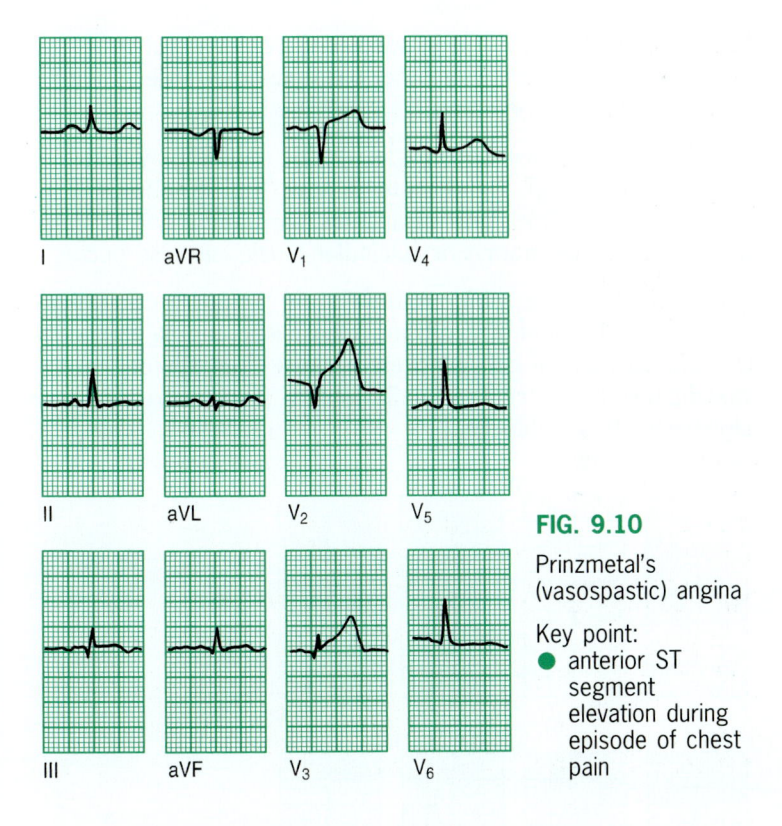

the spasm is superimposed upon some degree of atherosclerosis. Although any artery can be affected, spasm most commonly occurs in the right coronary artery. During an episode of vasospasm, the patient develops ST segment elevation in the affected territory (Fig. 9.10).

Although the combination of chest pain and ST segment elevation often suggests myocardial infarction, vasospastic angina is distinguished by the transient nature of the ST segment elevation. Unlike myocardial infarction, the ECG changes of vasospastic angina resolve entirely when the episode of chest pain settles. Ask the patient about a history of prior episodes of chest pain, which typically occur at rest

168 MAKING SENSE OF THE ECG

and particularly overnight in vasospastic angina. Patients may also have a history of other vasospastic disorders, such as Raynaud's phenomenon.

The ST segment elevation of vasospastic angina may be accompanied by tall 'hyperacute' T waves or, sometimes, T wave inversion. Transient intraventricular conduction defects, such as a bundle branch or fascicular block, can also occur.

Treatment for vasospastic angina should include a calcium-channel blocker and/or a nitrate. Vasospastic angina can worsen with use of beta blockers because they act on vasodilatory beta receptors while leaving vasoconstrictory alpha receptors unblocked.

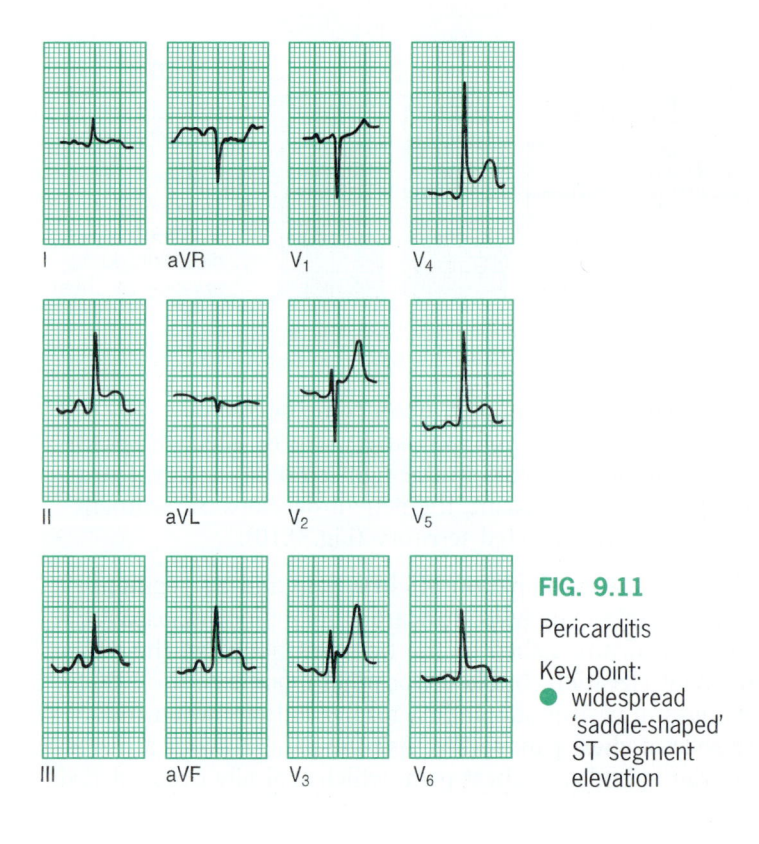

FIG. 9.11

Pericarditis

Key point:
- widespread 'saddle-shaped' ST segment elevation

Pericarditis

The ST segment elevation of pericarditis (Fig. 9.11) has four characteristics that, while not pathognomonic, help to distinguish it from acute myocardial infarction:

- The ST segment elevation is typically widespread, affecting all of those leads (anterolateral and inferior) which 'look at' the inflamed epicardium. Leads aVR and V_1 usually show reciprocal ST segment depression.
- The ST segment elevation is characteristically 'saddle shaped' (concave upward).
- T wave inversion occurs only *after* the ST segments have returned to baseline.
- Q waves do not develop.

The assessment of a patient with pericarditis should aim not only at confirming the diagnosis but also at establishing the cause (Table 9.3).

Clinically, the pain of pericarditis can usually be distinguished from that of myocardial infarction. Although both produce a retrosternal pain, that of pericarditis is sharp and pleuritic, exacerbated by inspiration and relieved by sitting forward. A friction rub on auscultation is pathognomonic of pericarditis.

Direct treatment of the underlying cause should be carried out where possible. Anti-inflammatory agents

Table 9.3 Causes of pericarditis

- Infectious
    - viral (e.g. Coxsackie)
    - bacterial (e.g. *Staphylococcus*)
    - tuberculous
- Myocardial infarction (first few days)
- Dressler's syndrome (1 month or more post-MI)
- Uraemia
- Malignancy
- Connective tissue disease
- Radiotherapy

FIG. 9.13

Myocardial ischaemia

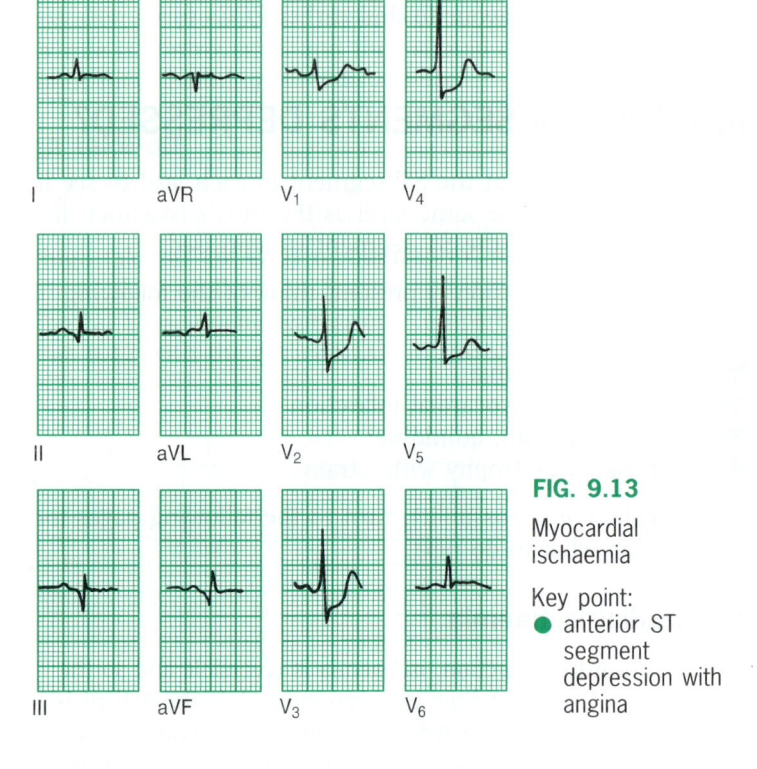

Key point:
- anterior ST segment depression with angina

The management of stable angina includes:

- modifying any risk factors (e.g. smoking, hypertension)
- aspirin, 150 mg once daily
- glyceryl trinitrate (GTN) sublingually as required.

Add in antianginal therapy as necessary to control symptoms:

- beta blocker
- calcium antagonist
- long-acting oral or transdermal nitrate.

If antianginal drugs fail to control symptoms adequately, go on to consider cardiac catheterization with a view to:

- percutaneous transluminal coronary angioplasty (PTCA)
- coronary artery bypass surgery.

Rapidly worsening chest pain, chest pain of recent onset or chest pain at rest indicates **unstable angina**. This is a medical emergency, with a 1-year mortality of up to 20% in untreated patients, so urgent treatment is essential. Initial treatment includes:

- bedrest
- analgesia
- aspirin
- beta blockers
- intravenous heparin
- intravenous nitrates.

If unstable angina does not settle with drug treatment, consider cardiac catheterization with a view to urgent intervention – discuss this with a cardiologist.

ACT QUICKLY

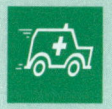

Unstable angina is a medical emergency. Prompt diagnosis and treatment are essential.

Acute posterior myocardial infarction

Acute posterior myocardial infarction was discussed in Chapter 8. It can cause ST segment depression in the chest leads V_1–V_3, together with:

- dominant R waves
- upright, tall T waves.

An example is shown in Fig. 8.4.

The management of posterior myocardial infarction is the same of that of other Q wave myocardial infarctions, as outlined earlier in this chapter.

9

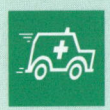

> **ACT QUICKLY**
>
> Acute myocardial infarction is a medical emergency. Prompt diagnosis and treatment are essential.

Drugs

Two antiarrhythmic drugs affect the ST segment:

- digoxin
- quinidine.

Digoxin has a characteristic effect on the ST segment, which is just one of a number of its effects on the whole ECG (Table 9.4). The ST segment depression seen with digoxin is described as a 'reverse tick', and is most obvious in leads with tall R waves (Fig. 9.14).

You must always distinguish between digoxin *effects*, which may be apparent at therapeutic doses, and digoxin *toxicity*, which indicates overdosage. If digoxin toxicity is a possibility, ask about symptoms (anorexia, nausea, vomiting, abdominal

Table 9.4 Effects of digoxin on the ECG

At therapeutic levels
- ST segment depression ('reverse tick')
- Reduction in T wave size
- Shortening of the QT interval

At toxic levels
- T wave inversion
- Arrhythmias – almost any, but especially:
    - sinus bradycardia
    - paroxysmal atrial tachycardia with block
    - atrioventricular block
    - ventricular ectopics
    - ventricular bigeminy
    - ventricular tachycardia

FIG. 9.14

Digoxin effect

Key point:
- 'reverse tick' ST segment depression

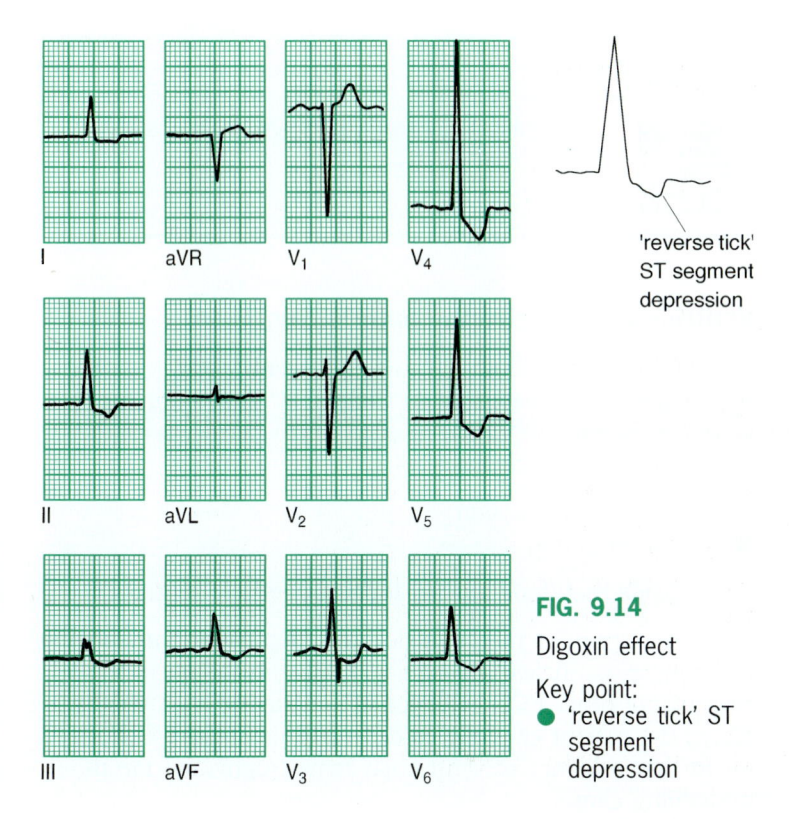

pain and visual disturbance) and check a digoxin level and plasma potassium level (arrhythmias are more likely if the patient is hypokalaemic).

Treat digoxin toxicity by stopping the drug and, where necessary, correcting potassium levels and treating arrhythmias. A digoxin-specific antibody may be used if the problem is life threatening, but should not be used without expert advice.

Quinidine also has a number of effects on the ECG, one of which is ST segment depression (which is *not* 'reverse tick' in character).

DRUG POINT

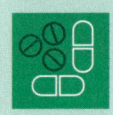

A complete drug history is essential in any patient with an abnormal ECG.

Ventricular hypertrophy with 'strain'

The appearances of both left and right ventricular hypertrophy were discussed in Chapter 8. The 'strain' pattern is said to be present when, in addition to tall R waves and deep S waves, there is also:

- ST segment depression
- T wave inversion

in the leads that 'look at' the affected ventricle (Fig. 9.15).

The term 'strain' is rather misleading, because the underlying mechanism is unclear. If you see T wave inversion in the presence of other ECG evidence of ventricular hypertrophy, assess the patient carefully as described in Chapter 8, both for further evidence of ventricular hypertrophy and for an underlying cause.

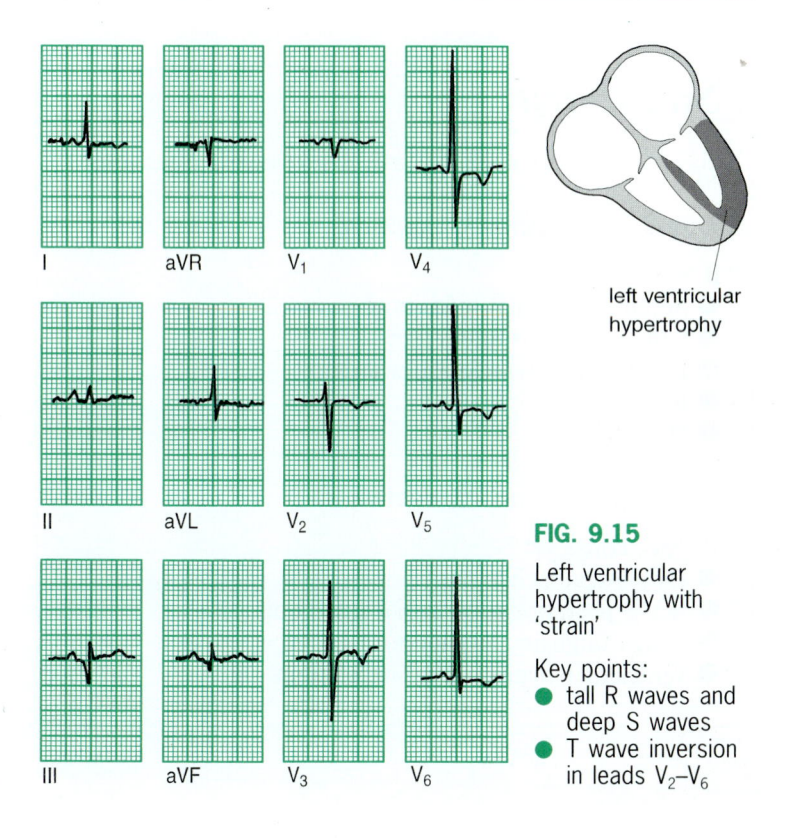

THE ST SEGMENT 177

I	aVR	V₁	V₄
II	aVL	V₂	V₅
III	aVF	V₃	V₆

left ventricular hypertrophy

FIG. 9.15

Left ventricular hypertrophy with 'strain'

Key points:
- tall R waves and deep S waves
- T wave inversion in leads V₂–V₆

Summary

To assess the ST segment, ask the following questions:

1. Are the ST segments elevated?

If 'yes', consider:
- Acute myocardial infarction
- Left ventricular aneurysm
- Prinzmetal's (vasospastic) angina
- Pericarditis
- High take-off

2. Are the ST segments depressed?

If 'yes', consider:
- Myocardial ischaemia
- Acute posterior myocardial infarction
- Drugs (digoxin, quinidine)
- Ventricular hypertrophy with 'strain'

10

THE T WAVE

After examining the ST segment, look carefully at the size and orientation of the T wave. The T wave corresponds to ventricular repolarization. The shape and orientation of normal T waves are shown in Fig. 10.1.

It is normal for the T wave to be inverted in lead aVR. In some cases, T wave inversion can also be normal in leads III, V_1 and V_2, and these occurrences are discussed later in this chapter.

T waves can be abnormal in one of three ways, so the questions you need to ask about them are:

- Are the T waves too tall?
- Are the T waves too small?
- Are any of the T waves inverted?

ARE THE T WAVES TOO TALL?

There is no clearly defined normal range for T wave height, although, as a general guide, a T wave should be no more than half the size of the preceding QRS complex. Your ability to recognize abnormally tall T waves will improve as you examine increasing numbers of ECGs and gain experience of the normal variations that occur.

If you suspect that the T waves are abnormally tall, consider whether your patient could have either of the following:

FIG. 10.1

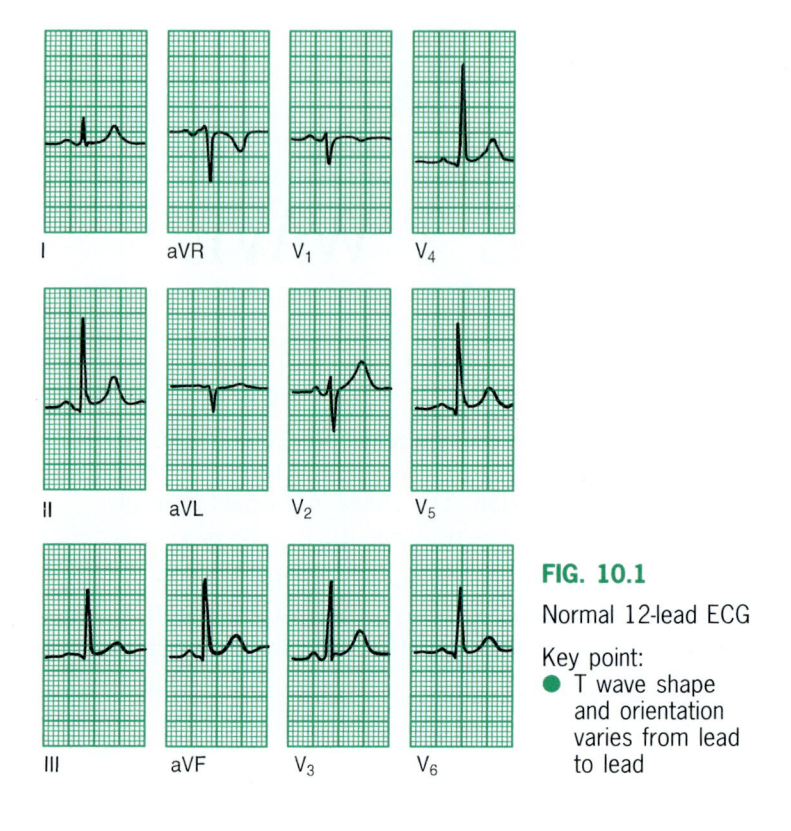

Normal 12-lead ECG

Key point:
- T wave shape and orientation varies from lead to lead

- hyperkalaemia
- acute myocardial infarction.

If either is a possibility, turn to the following pages for guidance on what to do next.

Bear in mind, however, that tall T waves are often just a variant of normal, especially if you are judging just a single ECG. Your level of suspicion should be higher, however, if you are comparing against earlier ECGs from the same patient and the height of the T waves has increased significantly.

THE T WAVE

FIG. 10.2

Hyperkalaemia

Key point:
- tall 'tented' T waves

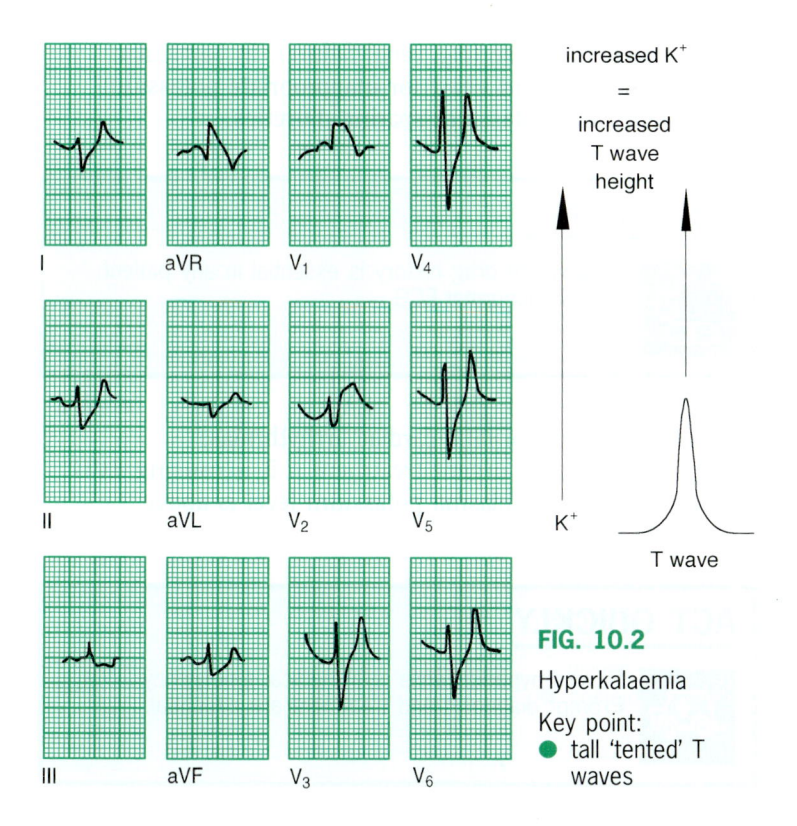

Hyperkalaemia

An elevated plasma potassium level can cause tall 'tented' T waves (Fig. 10.2). Hyperkalaemia may also widen the T waves so that the entire ST segment is incorporated into the upstroke of the T wave. Hyperkalaemia may also cause:

- flattening and even loss of the P wave
- lengthening of the PR interval
- widening of the QRS complex
- arrhythmias.

If the diagnosis is confirmed by an elevated plasma potassium level, assess the patient for symptoms and signs

ARE THE T WAVES TOO SMALL?

As with tall T waves, the judgement of whether T waves are abnormally small is rather subjective.

If you suspect that the T waves are abnormally small, consider whether your patient could have one of the following:

- hypokalaemia
- pericardial effusion
- hypothyroidism.

Advice about the diagnosis and treatment of each of these is given on the following pages.

Hypokalaemia

Just as hyperkalaemia causes tall T waves, so hypokalaemia causes small T waves (Fig. 10.4). Look carefully for other ECG changes that may accompany hypokalaemia:

- first-degree heart block
- depression of the ST segment
- prominent U waves.

If hypokalaemia is suspected, assess the patient for symptoms (e.g. muscle weakness, cramps) and review their treatment chart. Although a number of conditions lead to hypokalaemia, the commonest cause is diuretics.

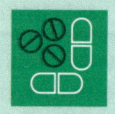

> **DRUG POINT**
>
> A complete drug history is essential in any patient with an abnormal ECG.

Check the plasma electrolytes to confirm the diagnosis. Oral potassium supplements are sufficient if the plasma potassium

THE T WAVE

FIG. 10.4

Hypokalaemia

Key points:
- small T waves
- prominent U waves

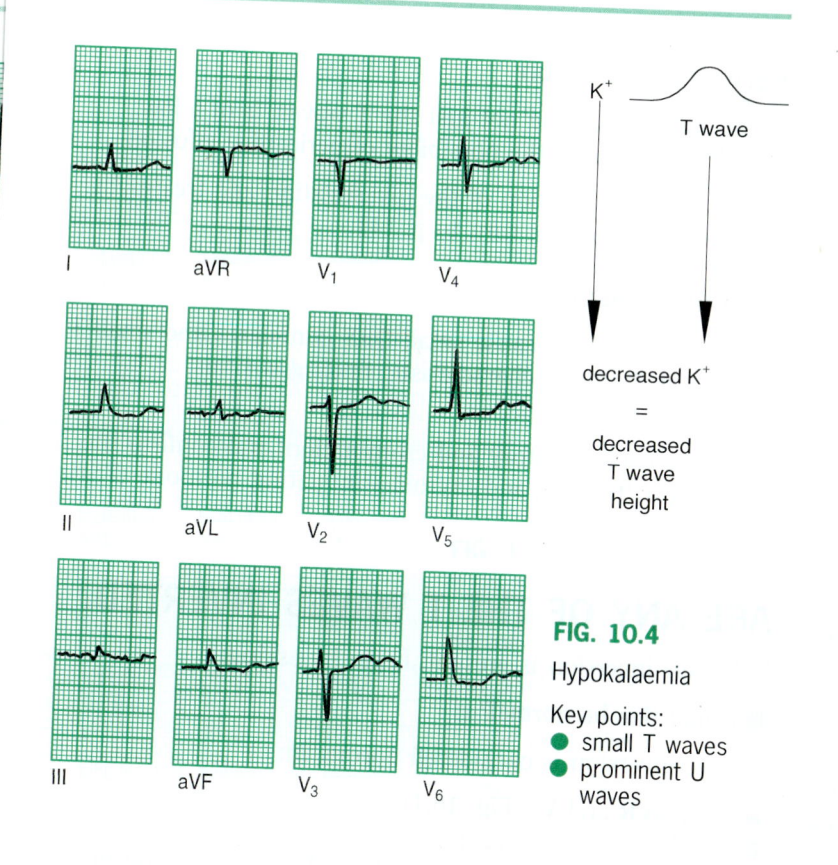

decreased K^+ = decreased T wave height

level is above 2.5 mmol/l and the patient is asymptomatic. More severe hypokalaemia, or the presence of symptoms, requires cautious correction with a slow intravenous infusion of potassium chloride.

ACT QUICKLY

Severe hypokalaemia is a medical emergency. Prompt diagnosis and treatment are essential.

- pericarditis (Chapter 9)
- permanent ventricular pacing (Chapter 14).

Finally, there are four conditions where T wave inversion can occur but the ECG is not diagnostic:

- hyperventilation
- mitral valve prolapse
- pulmonary embolism
- subarachnoid haemorrhage.

If your patient has one of these conditions, you do not need to look for another cause of T wave inversion without other reasons to suspect one.

Myocardial ischaemia

ST segment depression is the commonest manifestation of myocardial ischaemia (Chapter 9), but T wave inversion may also occur in the leads that 'look at' the affected areas (Fig. 10.6). Because ischaemia is reversible, these ECG abnormalities will only be observed during an ischaemic episode.

Patients whose T waves are inverted to begin with (e.g. following a myocardial infarction) may develop temporarily *upright* T waves during ischaemic episodes. This is referred to as T wave **'pseudonormalization'**.

The management of myocardial ischaemia is described in detail on p. 171.

Myocardial infarction

T wave inversion can occur not only as a temporary change in myocardial ischaemia, but also as a more prolonged (and sometimes permanent) change in myocardial infarction. In Chapter 9, we mentioned that myocardial infarctions are often divided into:

- Q wave infarcts
- non-Q wave infarcts.

T wave inversion can occur in either type of infarct – the defining characteristic is whether Q waves appear or not.

FIG. 10.6

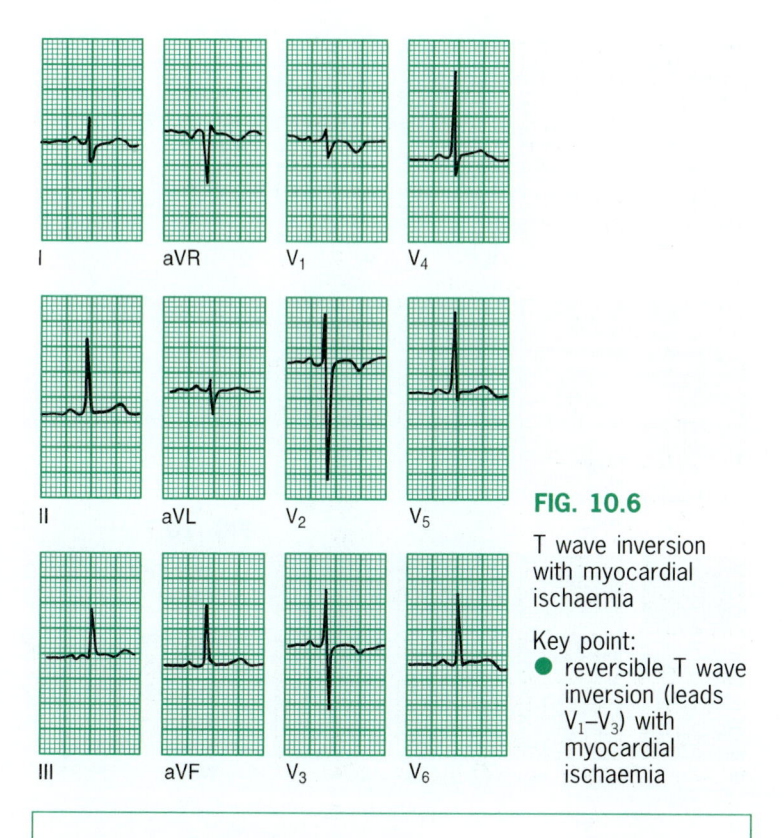

T wave inversion with myocardial ischaemia

Key point:
- reversible T wave inversion (leads V_1–V_3) with myocardial ischaemia

---

Q wave vs non-Q wave infarction

The suggestion that Q wave infarcts always involve the full thickness of the myocardium, while non-Q wave infarcts only involve the subendocardial region, is misleading. Post-mortem studies have shown that this distinction is often incorrect, and so the terms 'full thickness' and 'subendocardial' are probably better avoided.

So why make the distinction between Q wave and non-Q wave infarcts at all? It is important for two reasons. First, there is currently no definitive evidence that thrombolysis improves prognosis in non-Q wave infarction. Second, patients with non-Q wave infarction may be at higher risk of reinfarction than those presenting with Q wave infarcts, although there is no overall difference in 3-year mortality.

190 MAKING SENSE OF THE ECG

FIG. 10.7

Q wave myocardial infarction

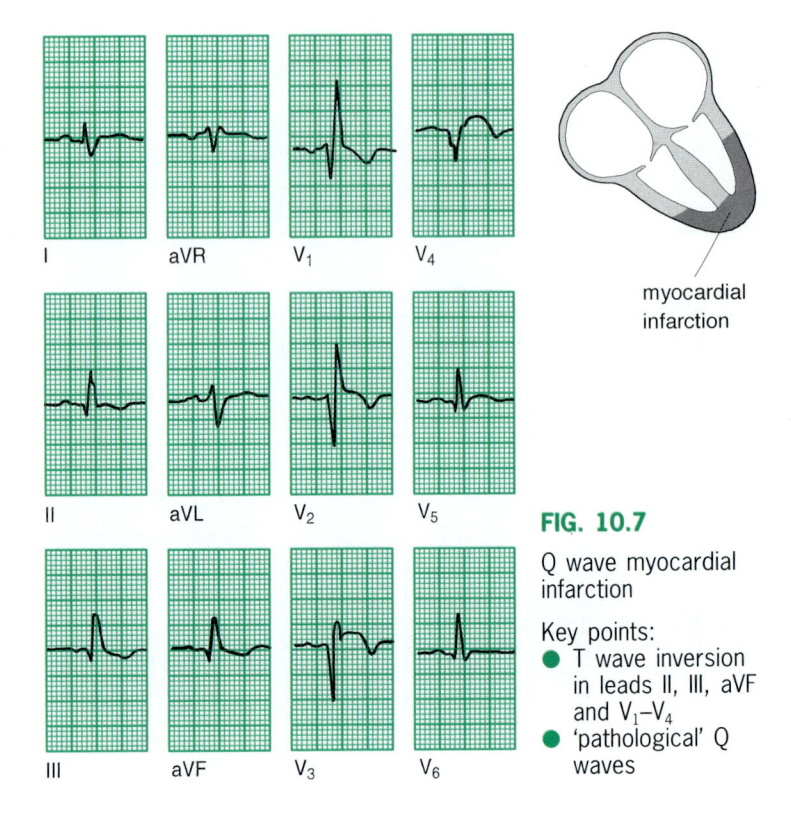

Key points:
- T wave inversion in leads II, III, aVF and V_1–V_4
- 'pathological' Q waves

In **Q wave infarction**, the T wave inversion accompanies the return of the elevated ST segment to baseline (Fig. 10.7). T wave inversion may be permanent, or the T wave may return to normal.

Non-Q wave infarction also causes T wave inversion (Fig. 10.8), although it can also manifest as ST segment depression alone.

If you see abnormal T wave inversion on an ECG, question the patient about any history of chest pain and previous angina or myocardial infarctions, and assess their risk factors for ischaemic heart disease (Table 9.1).

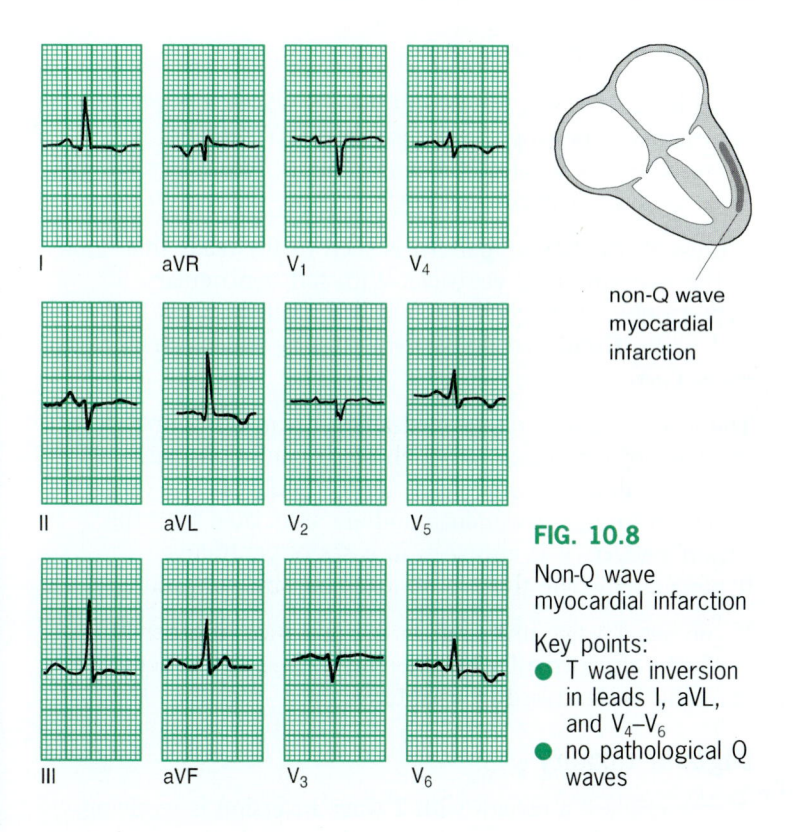

THE T WAVE

FIG. 10.8

Non-Q wave myocardial infarction

Key points:
- T wave inversion in leads I, aVL, and V_4–V_6
- no pathological Q waves

The management of Q wave myocardial infarction is detailed in Chapter 9.

ACT QUICKLY

Acute myocardial infarction is a medical emergency. Prompt diagnosis and treatment are essential.

Ventricular hypertrophy

In addition to tall R waves and deep S waves (Chapter 8), ventricular hypertrophy can also cause ST segment depression and T wave inversion. This is commonly referred to as a 'strain' pattern (p. 176).

If present, the 'strain' pattern is seen in the leads that 'look' at the hypertrophied ventricle. With **left** ventricular hypertrophy the abnormalities will be seen in leads I, aVL and V_4–V_6. **Right** ventricular hypertrophy causes changes in leads V_1–V_3.

The term 'strain' is rather misleading because the underlying mechanism is unclear. Although some conditions, such as massive pulmonary embolism, can certainly place a ventricle under an increased workload and are associated with the 'strain' pattern, it is also seen in cases of ventricular hypertrophy where there is no apparent stress on the ventricle.

If you see T wave inversion in the presence of other ECG evidence of ventricular hypertrophy, assess the patient carefully as described in Chapter 8.

Digoxin toxicity

Always check if a patient with T wave inversion is receiving treatment with digoxin, as this can be an indication of digoxin toxicity (Fig. 10.9). This is just one of a number of ECG changes that can be seen in patients taking digoxin (Table 9.4).

The diagnosis and treatment of digoxin toxicity are covered in more detail on p. 174.

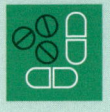

> **DRUG POINT**
>
> A complete drug history is essential in any patient with an abnormal ECG.

THE T WAVE 193

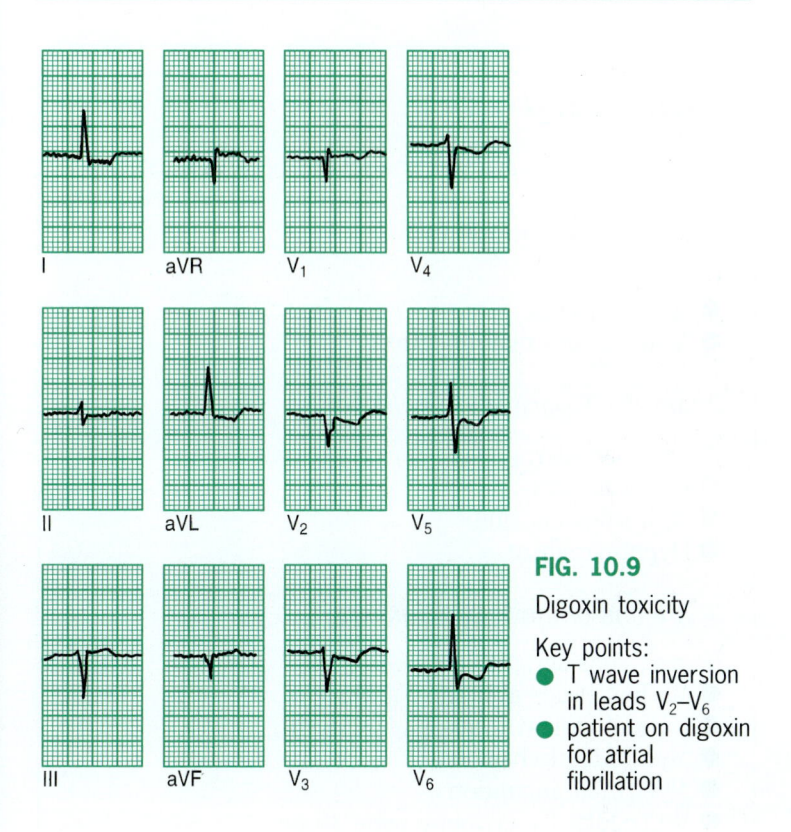

FIG. 10.9

Digoxin toxicity

Key points:
- T wave inversion in leads V_2–V_6
- patient on digoxin for atrial fibrillation

Summary

To assess the T wave, ask the following questions:

1. Are the T waves too tall?

If 'yes', consider:
- Hyperkalaemia
- Acute myocardial infarction

2. Are the T waves too small?

If 'yes', consider:
- Hypokalaemia
- Pericardial effusion
- Hypothyroidism

3. Are any of the T waves inverted?

If 'yes', consider:
- Normal (leads aVR and V_1)
- Normal variant (leads V_2, V_3 and III)
- Myocardial ischaemia
- Myocardial infarction
- Ventricular hypertrophy with 'strain'
- Digoxin toxicity

Also bear in mind:

- Following paroxysmal tachycardia (Chapter 3)
- Bundle branch block (Chapter 8)
- Pericarditis (Chapter 9)
- Permanent ventricular pacing (Chapter 14)
- Hyperventilation
- Mitral valve prolapse
- Pulmonary embolism
- Subarachnoid haemorrhage

11

THE QT INTERVAL

After examining the T waves, measure the QT interval. This is the time from the *start* of the QRS complex to the *end* of the T wave (Fig. 11.1), and it represents the total duration of electrical activity (depolarization and repolarization) in the ventricles.

When determining the duration of the QT interval, it is important to measure it to the end of the T wave and not

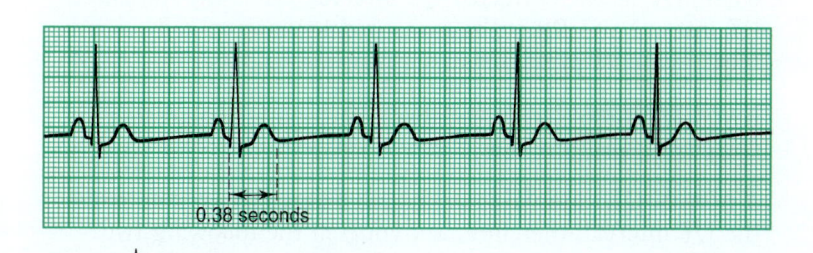

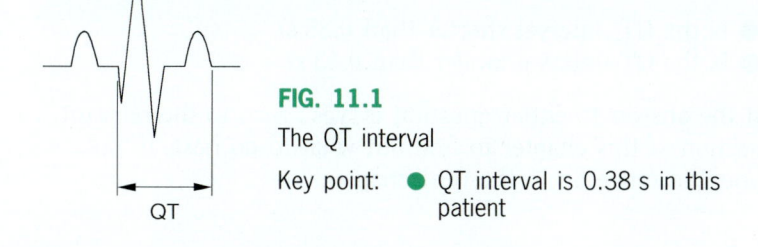

FIG. 11.1

The QT interval

Key point: ● QT interval is 0.38 s in this patient

196 MAKING SENSE OF THE ECG

the U wave (if one is present – see Chapter 12). Mistaking a U wave for a T wave is easily done and overestimates the QT interval. To reduce the likelihood of this, measure the QT interval in lead aVL, where U waves are least prominent.

As with any interval in the ECG, there are only two possible abnormalities of the QT interval:

- The QT interval can be too long.
- The QT interval can be too short.

Unfortunately, deciding whether or not the QT interval is normal is not entirely straightforward, because the duration varies according to the patient's heart rate: the faster the heart rate the shorter the QT interval. To allow for this, you must calculate the corrected QT interval (QT_c) using the following formula:

$$QT_c = \frac{QT}{\sqrt{RR}}$$

where QT_c is the corrected QT interval, QT is the measured QT interval and RR is the measured RR interval (all measurements in seconds).

If you are interested in the theory behind QT interval correction, read the box.

A normal QT_c interval is 0.35–0.43 s long. When you assess the QT interval, therefore, ask yourself the following two questions:

- Is the QT_c interval shorter than 0.35 s?
- Is the QT_c interval longer than 0.43 s?

If the answer to either question is 'yes', turn to the relevant section of this chapter to find out what to do next. If 'no', you can move on to the next chapter.

Why correct the QT interval?

Correction of the QT interval is necessary because the normal QT interval varies with heart rate: the faster the heart rate, the shorter the normal QT interval. Although graphs and tables of normal QT intervals at different heart rates are available, it is inconvenient to have to look up the normal range every time you want to check someone's QT interval.

A much better way to assess a QT interval is to correct it to what it *would* be if the patient's heart rate was 60 beats per minute. By doing this, all you will then need to remember is *one* normal range for the QT interval.

You will need a pocket calculator to calculate the corrected QT interval ('QT_c interval'). Divide the patient's measured QT interval (measured in seconds) by the square root of their RR interval (also measured in seconds). This is Bazett's formula:

$$QT_c = \frac{QT}{\sqrt{RR}}$$

The RR interval is the time between consecutive R waves, and can be either measured directly from the ECG or calculated by dividing 60 by the patient's heart rate. For example, at a heart rate of 80 beats per minute the RR interval is 0.75 s.

Many of the more sophisticated ECG machines automatically print out a value for the QT_c interval on the ECG. However, always check for yourself values that are automatically measured in this way as errors do occur.

The normal range for the QT interval at a heart rate of 60 beats per minute, and thus for the QT_c interval, is from 0.35 s to 0.43 s.

IS THE QT_C INTERVAL SHORTER THAN 0.35 SECONDS?

If the answer is 'yes', your patient's corrected QT interval is shorter than normal and you should check for the following:

- hypercalcaemia
- digoxin effect.

If either of these is a possibility, read the following pages to find out what to do next.

Shortening of the QT$_c$ interval is also recognized in:

- hyperthermia.

Having established the diagnosis of hyperthermia clinically, you will not need to look for another cause for a shortened QT$_c$ interval without a good reason to do so.

Hypercalcaemia

The shortened QT interval in hypercalcaemia results from abnormally rapid ventricular repolarization (Fig. 11.2).

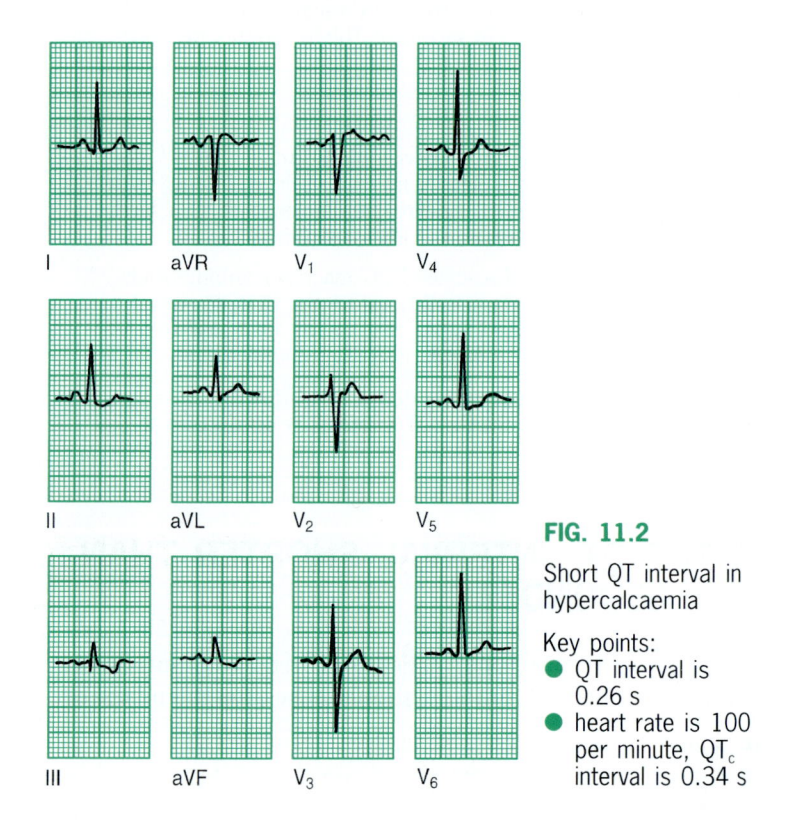

FIG. 11.2

Short QT interval in hypercalcaemia

Key points:
- QT interval is 0.26 s
- heart rate is 100 per minute, QT$_c$ interval is 0.34 s

Symptoms of hypercalcaemia include anorexia, weight loss, nausea, vomiting, abdominal pain, constipation, polydipsia, polyuria, weakness and depression.

A prominent U wave (Chapter 12) may also be seen in hypercalcaemia. Confirm the diagnosis with a plasma calcium level (correcting the result for the patient's current albumin level). The underlying causes that you need to consider are listed in Table 11.1.

Table 11.1 Causes of hypercalcaemia

- Hyperparathyroidism
  - primary
  - tertiary
- Malignancy (including myeloma)
- Drugs
  - thiazide diuretics
  - excessive vitamin D intake
- Sarcoidosis
- Thyrotoxicosis
- Milk-alkali syndrome

The treatment of hypercalcaemia depends, in the long term, on the underlying cause. Immediate management depends upon the symptoms and plasma calcium level. There is a risk of cardiac arrest with severe hypercalcaemia, so prompt recognition and treatment are essential.

Severe symptoms (e.g. vomiting, drowsiness) or a plasma calcium level greater than 3.5 mmol/l warrant urgent treatment as follows:

- intravenous 0.9% saline (e.g. 3–4 l per 24 h)
- intravenous frusemide (20–40 mg every 6–12 h *after rehydration*)
- bisphosphonates (e.g. disodium pamidronate – single infusion of 30 mg over 2 h)

202 MAKING SENSE OF THE ECG

FIG. 11.3

Long QT interval in hypocalcaemia

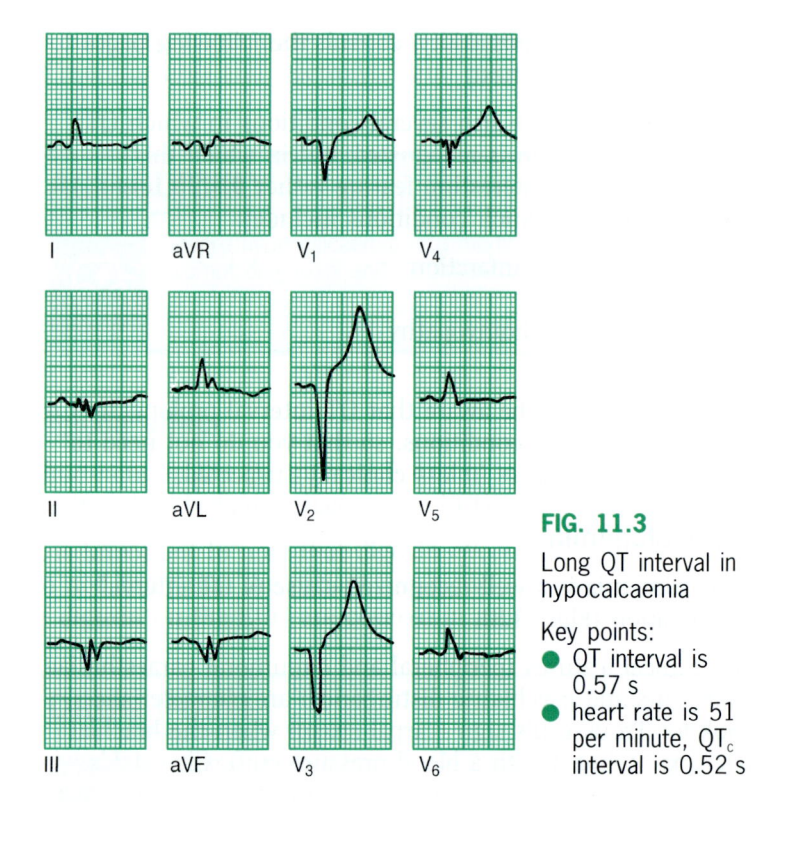

Key points:
- QT interval is 0.57 s
- heart rate is 51 per minute, QT_c interval is 0.52 s

Table 11.2 Causes of hypocalcaemia

- Hypoparathyroidism
  - following thyroid surgery
  - autoimmune
  - congenital (DiGeorge syndrome)
- Pseudohypoparathyroidism
- Chronic renal failure
- Vitamin D deficiency/resistance
- Drugs (e.g. calcitonin)
- Acute pancreatitis

monitor plasma calcium levels to avoid overtreatment and consequent hypercalcaemia.

Drug effects

A number of antiarrhythmic drugs cause prolongation of the QT interval by slowing myocardial conduction, and thus repolarization. Examples include quinidine, procainamide and flecainide. QT interval prolongation is also seen with tricyclic antidepressants.

Drug-induced QT interval prolongation is associated with torsades de pointes (Chapter 3) which can lead to ventricular fibrillation and sudden cardiac death. The problem therefore requires immediate attention, and referral to a cardiologist for review of antiarrhythmic drug treatment is recommended.

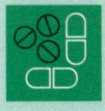

> **DRUG POINT**
>
> A complete drug history is essential in any patient with an abnormal ECG.

Acute myocarditis

QT interval prolongation can occur with any cause of acute myocarditis, although it is most usually associated with rheumatoid carditis.

Presenting features often include a fever, chest discomfort, palpitations and symptoms of heart failure (dyspnoea and fatigue). Examination may reveal quiet heart sounds, a friction rub, tachycardia, a fourth heart sound and gallop rhythm. There may also be features specific to the underlying cause (Table 11.3).

Table 11.3 Causes of myocarditis

- Infectious
  - viral (e.g. Coxsackie, influenza)
  - bacterial (e.g. acute rheumatic fever, diphtheria)
  - protozoal (e.g. Chagas' disease, toxoplasmosis)
  - rickettsial
- Drug-induced (e.g. chloroquine)
- Toxic agents (e.g. lead)
- Peripartum

Other ECG changes may be present, including:

- ST segment changes
- T wave inversion
- heart block (of any degree of severity)
- arrhythmias.

A chest X-ray may show cardiomegaly. A cardiac biopsy reveals acute inflammatory changes, and the levels of cardiac enzymes will be raised. Rarely, viral serology may establish the aetiology.

The treatment of acute myocarditis is supportive. Bedrest is recommended. Treat heart failure, arrhythmias and heart block as necessary. Antibiotics are indicated where a responsive organism is suspected. Although many patients will go on to make a good recovery, some are left with heart failure.

SEEK HELP

Acute myocarditis requires specialist assessment. Obtain the advice of a cardiologist without delay.

Hereditary syndromes

Prolongation of the QT interval occurs in two hereditary syndromes:

- Jervill and Lange-Nielsen syndrome
- Romano–Ward syndrome.

The autosomal recessive Jervill and Lange-Nielsen syndrome consists of congenital high-tone deafness, recurrent syncopal attacks and sudden death secondary to ventricular tachycardia, torsades de pointes and ventricular fibrillation. The arrhythmias are often triggered by exercise or stress.

The autosomal dominant Romano–Ward syndrome carries the same risk of ventricular arrhythmias but hearing is normal.

Prolonged QT intervals may be detected incidentally on an ECG in an asymptomatic individual, or in a patient presenting with a ventricular arrhythmia. Although rare, both syndromes are associated with torsades de pointes (Chapter 3) and sudden cardiac death. Referral to a cardiologist is recommended.

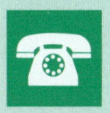

> **SEEK HELP**
>
> Hereditary long-QT syndromes are life threatening. Obtain the advice of a cardiologist without delay.

Summary

To assess the QT interval, ask the following questions:

1. Is the QT_c interval shorter than 0.35 s?

If 'yes', consider:
- Hypercalcaemia
- Digoxin effect (p. 174)

Also bear in mind:

- Hyperthermia

2. Is the QT_c interval longer than 0.43 s?

If 'yes', consider:
- Hypocalcaemia
- Drug effects
- Acute myocarditis
- Hereditary syndromes

Also bear in mind:

- Acute myocardial infarction (p. 156)
- Cerebral injury
- Hypertrophic cardiomyopathy
- Hypothermia

12

THE U WAVE

The U wave follows the T wave (Fig. 12.1) and is commonly seen in normal ECGs, although it can be

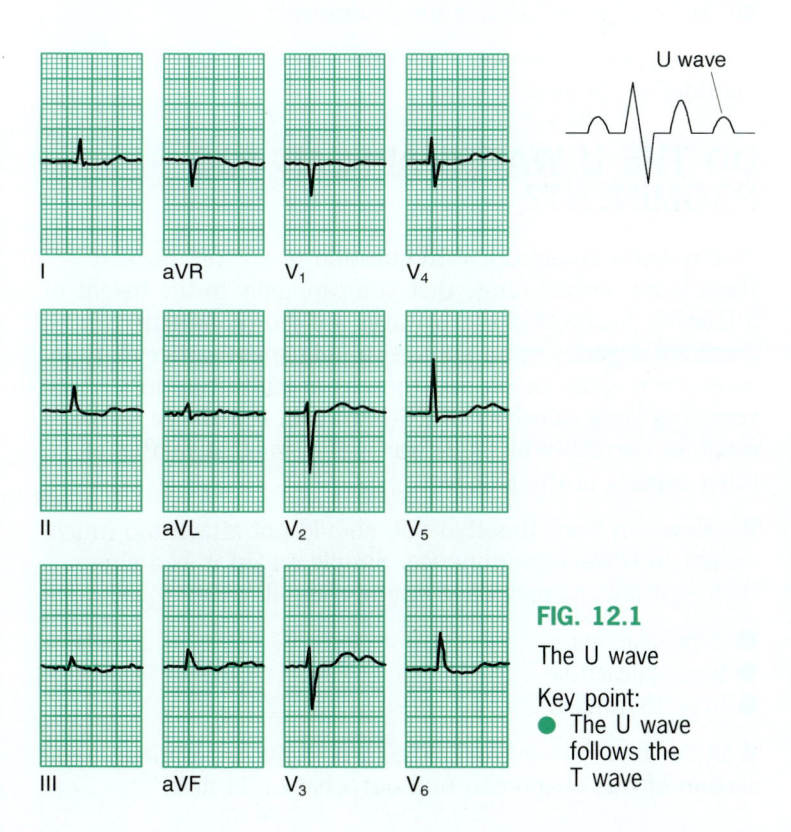

FIG. 12.1

The U wave

Key point:
- The U wave follows the T wave

difficult to discern clearly. When present, U waves are most clearly seen in the anterior chest leads V_2–V_4.

Although it is suggested that the U wave is caused by repolarization of the interventricular septum, this is by no means certain.

Normally, U waves are small and point in the same direction as the preceding T wave. Therefore, inverted U waves usually follow inverted T waves, and result from the same clinical abnormality (see Chapter 10).

U waves can also be abnormal in their own right, so when you assess the U wave, ask the following question:

● Do the U waves appear too prominent?

If the answer is 'yes', you will find a list of causes to consider in the next section.

DO THE U WAVES APPEAR TOO PROMINENT?

This is not a straightforward question to answer, because there is no normal range that you can apply to the height of a U wave. Suspecting the U waves are too prominent therefore depends upon subjective judgement rather than an objective measurement, and there is no substitute for reporting large numbers of ECGs to gain experience of the range of normality of the U wave (and, for that matter, all other aspects of the ECG).

It follows on from this that you should not attach too much weight to U wave prominence. Simply regard it as a clue that your patient may have one of the following:

● hypokalaemia
● hypercalcaemia
● hyperthyroidism.

If any of these are a possibility, turn to the appropriate section of this chapter to find out what to do next.

Hypokalaemia

Prominent U waves can be just one of a number of ECG abnormalities seen in the hypokalaemic patient (Fig. 12.2). Other associated ECG changes include:

- first-degree AV block (Chapter 6)
- depression of the ST segment (Chapter 9)
- small T waves (Chapter 10).

The investigation and treatment of hypokalaemia are discussed in detail on p. 181.

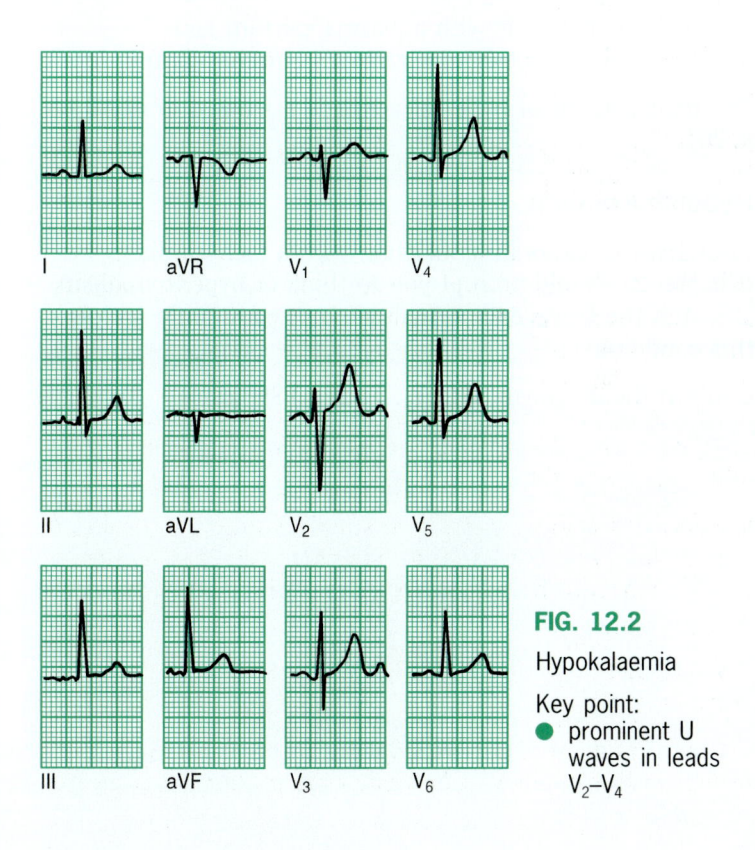

FIG. 12.2

Hypokalaemia

Key point:
- prominent U waves in leads V_2–V_4

ACT QUICKLY

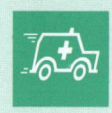

Severe hypokalaemia is a medical emergency. Prompt diagnosis and treatment are essential.

Hypercalcaemia

Always think of hypercalcaemia if you see prominent U waves, although hypercalcaemia is more characteristically associated with shortening of the QT interval (Chapter 11).

Confirm the diagnosis with a plasma calcium level (correcting the result for the patient's current albumin level).

The management of hypercalcaemia is discussed in detail on p. 201.

Hyperthyroidism

Prominent U waves in association with a tachycardia (Chapter 2) should prompt you to think of hyperthyroidism, although the U wave abnormality is not commonly seen in this condition.

Confirm the diagnosis with T_3, T_4 and TSH levels.

Summary

To assess the U wave, ask the following question:

1. Do the U waves appear too prominent?

If 'yes', consider:
- Hypokalaemia
- Hypercalcaemia
- Hyperthyroidism

Note: U waves can also be inverted, but this usually accompanies T wave inversion, the causes of which are discussed in Chapter 10.

13

ARTEFACTS ON THE ECG

If you encounter ECG abnormalities which appear atypical or which do not fit with the patient's clinical condition, always consider the possibility that they may be artefacts caused by:

- electrode misplacement
- external electrical interference
- incorrect calibration
- incorrect paper speed
- patient movement.

Examples of each of these are discussed on the following pages.

> **Remember**
> - Never give undue weight to a single investigation, particularly if the result does not fit with your clinical findings.
> - Do not hesitate to repeat an ECG if you suspect that the abnormalities could be artefacts.

ELECTRODE MISPLACEMENT

How to position correctly each recording electrode was discussed in Chapter 1. It can be quite easy to inadvertently

214 MAKING SENSE OF THE ECG

FIG. 13.1

Electrode misplacement

Key point:
- the left and right arm electrodes have been swapped over

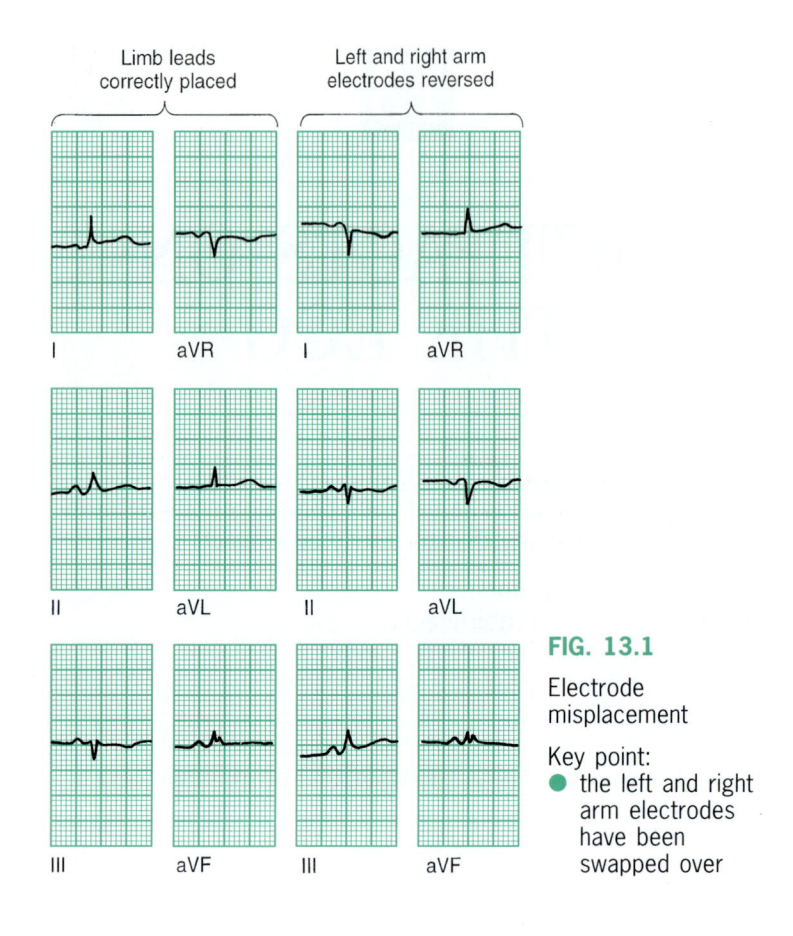

swap two electrodes over, and this is particularly common with the limb electrodes.

Figure 13.1 shows an ECG recorded with the two arm electrodes swapped over.

The abnormalities can be quite subtle, but you should always think of electrode misplacement if you see unexpected wave inversions.

EXTERNAL ELECTRICAL INTERFERENCE

External electrical interference (e.g. from electrical appliances) seldom causes difficulties when recording ECGs in hospital.

However, for general practitioners who sometimes record ECGs in patient's homes, 50 Hz electrical interference from domestic appliances has been reported as a significant cause of ECG artefact, and this can make the ECG difficult or even impossible to interpret correctly.

Always bear this in mind when interpreting an ECG recorded in a patient's home. Unless the source of the interference can be identified and removed, there is little that can be done apart from repeating the recording with the patient in a new location.

INCORRECT CALIBRATION

The standard ECG is recorded so that a voltage of 1 mV makes the recording needle move 10 mm. Every ECG must include a calibration mark (Fig. 13.2) so that the gain setting can be checked.

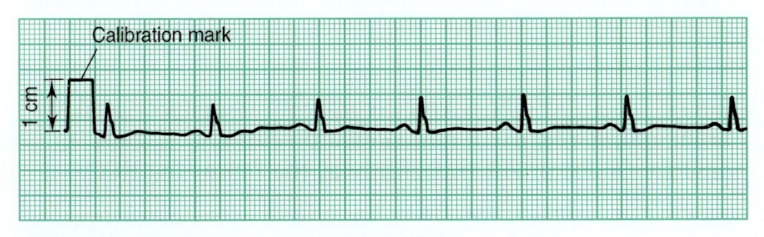

FIG. 13.2

Correct calibration

Key points:
- note 1 cm calibration mark
- 1 mV = 1 cm

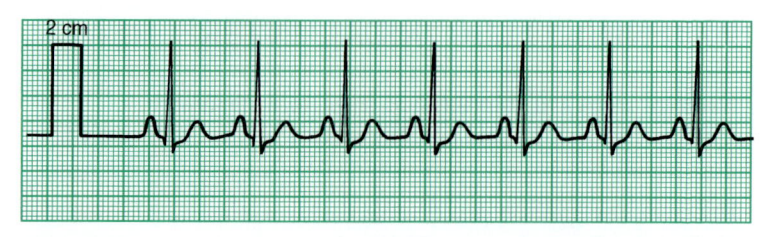

FIG. 13.3
Incorrect calibration
Key point: ● 1 mV = 2 cm

Sometimes it is necessary to alter the gain setting, particularly if the QRS complexes are so big at the standard setting that they will not fit clearly on the paper. If it is necessary to change to a non-standard calibration, it is good practice to record this clearly by writing a note on the ECG. If you see waves which appear too big or too small, always double check the size of the calibration mark (Fig. 13.3)

INCORRECT PAPER SPEED

In the UK and USA, the standard ECG recording speed is 25 mm/s, so that 1 small (1 mm) square equals 0.04 s. If the paper is run at double the speed (50 mm/s, which is standard in some parts of Europe), the waves will double in width (Fig. 13.4).

Always label every ECG you record with the paper speed used, and, if you use a non-standard setting, it is good practice to document this clearly at the top of the ECG.

PATIENT MOVEMENT

The ECG records the electrical activity of the heart, but this is not the only source of electrical activity in the body.

FIG. 13.4

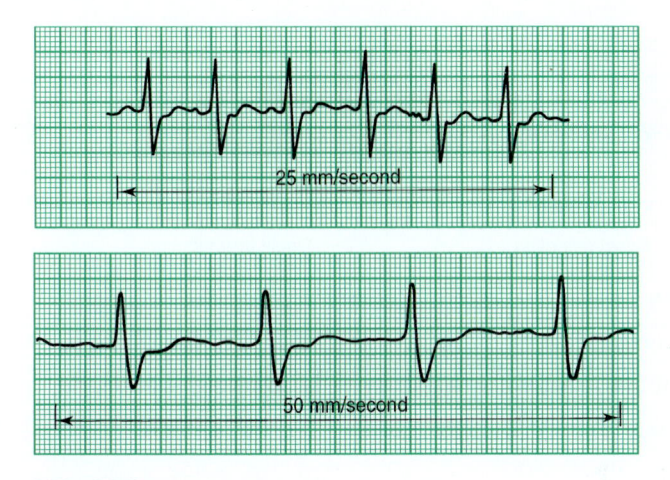

Incorrect paper speed

Key point: ● waves are abnormally wide at higher paper speeds

Skeletal muscle activity is also picked up on the ECG, and it is important for patients to lie still and relaxed while their ECG is recorded.

Unfortunately, this is not always possible, particularly if the patient is:

- uncooperative or agitated
- in respiratory distress
- suffering from a movement disorder.

Skeletal muscle activity is unavoidable during exercise testing. The use of signal-averaged ECGs, which 'average out' random electrical artefacts by combining a number of PQRST complexes, can help (Fig. 13.5). However, signal-averaged recordings can also be misleading by introducing artefactual changes of their own, and such recordings should always be interpreted with discretion.

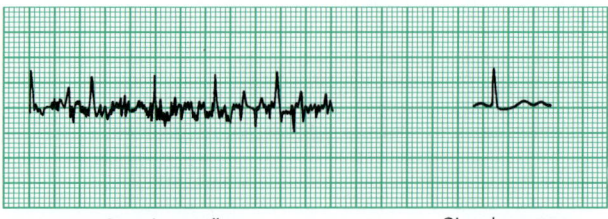

Actual recording　　　Signal average

FIG. 13.5

Signal-averaged ECG

Key point: ● electrical artefacts are reduced by signal averaging

---

Summary

For any ECG abnormality, always ask yourself:

1. Could this be artefactual?

If 'yes', consider:
- Electrode misplacement
- External electrical interference
- Incorrect calibration
- Incorrect paper speed
- Patient movement

14

PACEMAKERS

It is beyond the scope of this handbook to provide a detailed discussion of pacemakers. However, we have included a brief overview in this chapter for two reasons:

- Pacing is a treatment for a number of the abnormalities described in this book.
- Pacing affects the appearance of the ECG.

On the following pages you will find a general description of what pacemakers do, together with their indications.

WHAT DO PACEMAKERS DO?

Rapid advances in pacemaker technology have led to a remarkable increase in pacemaker sophistication, such that a wide range of different functions are now available. The most basic function of a pacemaker is to provide a 'safety net' in patients at risk of bradycardia. However, pacemakers that can terminate tachycardias are also available.

Pacemakers can either be **temporary**, to provide pacing in an emergency, or to tide patients over a short period of bradycardia (e.g. during a myocardial infarction) or until a permanent pacemaker can be implanted; or they can be **permanent**, in which case the battery, electronics and electrode(s) are all implanted within the patient. Temporary pacemakers are usually transvenous, but transoesophageal and transcutaneous pacing can also be used.

Patients seldom need pacing all the time, so both temporary and permanent pacemakers can be set up to monitor the heart's activity and only provide impulses when necessary. In the case of permanent pacemakers this is an effective way of prolonging the lifetime of the battery, typically to between 7 and 15 years.

INDICATIONS FOR TEMPORARY PACING

Patients awaiting permanent pacing

If patients have a severely symptomatic bradycardia but permanent pacing cannot be undertaken within an acceptable time, temporary pacing may be used to support them in the interim.

Acute myocardial infarction

In acute **inferior** myocardial infarction, damage to the artery that supplies the AV node can cause complete heart block and bradycardia. Few patients need help with temporary pacing, as blood pressure is usually maintained despite the slow heart rate. Temporary pacing is needed in second- and third-degree AV block with symptoms or haemodynamic disturbance.

Acute **anterior** myocardial infarction often causes hypotension as a result of damage to the left ventricle. Extensive infarction may involve the bundle branches in the interventricular septum and cause bradycardia. Mortality is high. Temporary pacing and inotropic support are necessary for second- and third-degree AV block, even when the condition is asymptomatic.

Tachycardia

Some tachycardias (including AV re-entry tachycardia and ventricular tachycardia) can be terminated by overdrive pacing. This should only be undertaken under the guidance of someone experienced in the technique – contact a cardiologist for assistance.

Perioperative pacing

See p. 225 for further information.

TEMPORARY PACEMAKER INSERTION AND CARE

Once the decision to insert a temporary pacemaker has been made, you must ensure that:

- the pacing wire is inserted using aseptic technique by a trained member of staff;
- X-ray screening time is kept to a minimum;
- a 'breathable' dressing is applied to the wound;
- a chest X-ray is ordered (and looked at!) after the pacemaker insertion to check for pneumothorax;
- the function of the pacemaker is monitored daily by checking the pacing threshold and ensuring the output is set at double the threshold;
- the pacing wire does not become dislodged;
- the pacing wire is removed at the earliest opportunity to prevent infection;
- the pacing wire is replaced, if still required, after 5 days, after which time infection risk increases sharply;
- temporary pacing is not withheld in acute myocardial infarction because of thrombolysis (the external jugular, brachiocephalic or femoral veins can be used for intravenous access routes in these circumstances, as these are superficial and easily compressed to control bleeding).

INDICATIONS FOR PERMANENT PACING

The decision to implant a *permanent* pacemaker must be made by a cardiologist, and you should seek their advice if you are uncertain about referring a patient. Generally speaking, the indications for a permanent pacemaker are:

- **Third-degree AV block** with an episode of syncope or presyncope. Asymptomatic patients with acquired third-degree AV block and a ventricular rate less than 40 beats per minute, or pauses greater than 3 s, should also be considered for pacing for prognostic reasons. Those with congenital third-degree AV block generally do not require pacing if they are asymptomatic, although they must be kept under regular review.
- **Second-degree AV block**, regardless of whether it is Mobitz type I or II, with an episode of symptomatic bradycardia.
- **Bi- or trifascicular block** with a clear history of syncope, or documented intermittent failure of the remaining fascicle.
- **Sick sinus syndrome** causing symptomatic bradycardia. Pacing is not usually necessary for asymptomatic patients.
- **Malignant vasovagal syndrome** is helped by pacing only if it is of the 'cardioinhibitory' variety which causes a bradycardia.
- **Carotid sinus syndrome** is also only helped by pacing when it is of the cardioinhibitory variety associated with a bradycardia.

SELECTION OF A PERMANENT PACEMAKER

A wide choice of permanent pacemakers is now available, each offering a different pacing strategy. The cardiologist will be responsible for selecting the most appropriate type of unit to be inserted, as well as providing long-term follow-up.

There is an internationally accepted code of up to five letters to describe the type of pacemaker. Each letter describes an aspect of the pacemaker's function, as outlined in Table 14.1.

Table 14.1 Pacemaker codes

Letter	Refers to	Code	Meaning
1	Chamber(s) paced	A V D	Atrium Ventricle Dual (both chambers)
2	Chamber(s) sensed	A V D O	Atrium Ventricle Dual (both chambers) None
3	Response to sensing	I T D O	Inhibition of pacemaker Triggering of pacemaker Inhibition or triggering None
4	Rate response	R	Rate-responsive pacemaker
5	Antitachycardia functions	P S D O	Pacing of tachycardias Shock delivered Dual (pacing and shock) None

Some of the most commonly encountered pacemakers are:

- **VVI** – this pacemaker has a single lead that senses activity in the ventricle. If no activity is detected, the pacemaker will take over control of the rhythm by pacing the ventricle via the same lead.
- **AAI** – this pacemaker also has a single lead, which is implanted in the atrium. It monitors atrial (P wave) activity. If normal atrial activity is not detected, it takes over by pacing the atria.
- **DDD** – this system has leads in both the atrium and the ventricle ('dual chamber'). It can both sense and pace via either lead. If it senses atrial activity but no ventricular activity, it will start pacing the ventricles in sequence with the atria. It can also pace the atria alone or, if AV conduction is blocked, pace the atria and ventricles sequentially.
- **AAIR, VVIR and DDDR** – the 'R' indicates that the pacemaker is rate responsive (see box).

Rate responsiveness

A rate-responsive pacemaker adjusts its pacing rate according to the patient's level of activity to mimic the physiological response to exercise. There are several parameters that can be monitored by pacemakers to determine the patient's level of activity, including vibration, respiration and blood temperature.

PACING AND THE ECG

Pacemakers activate depolarization with electrical impulses, and these appear as pacing 'spikes' on the ECG (Fig. 14.1). In ventricular pacing, a pacing spike will be followed by a broad QRS complex (because the depolarization is not conducted by the normal, fast-conduction pathways).

When the atria are being paced via an atrial lead, the pacing spike will be followed by a P wave. This may be conducted normally via the AV junction and be followed by a normal

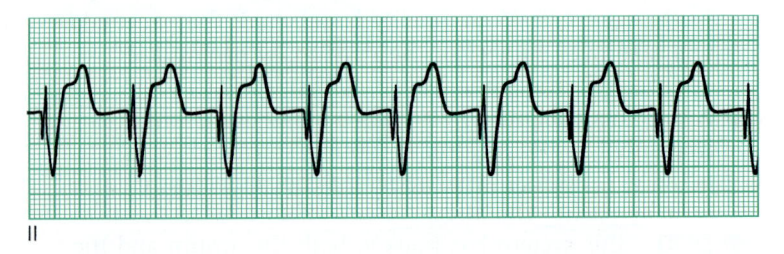

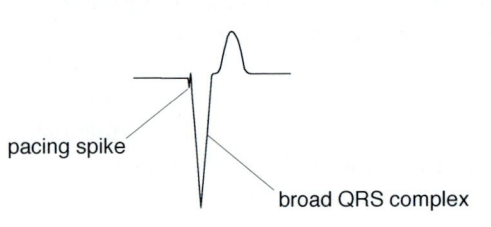

FIG. 14.1

Ventricular pacing

Key point:
- ventricular pacing spikes are followed by broad QRS complexes

FIG. 14.2

Dual chamber sequential pacing

Key points:
- atrial pacing spikes (large) are followed by inverted P waves
- ventricular pacing spikes (small) are followed by broad QRS complexes

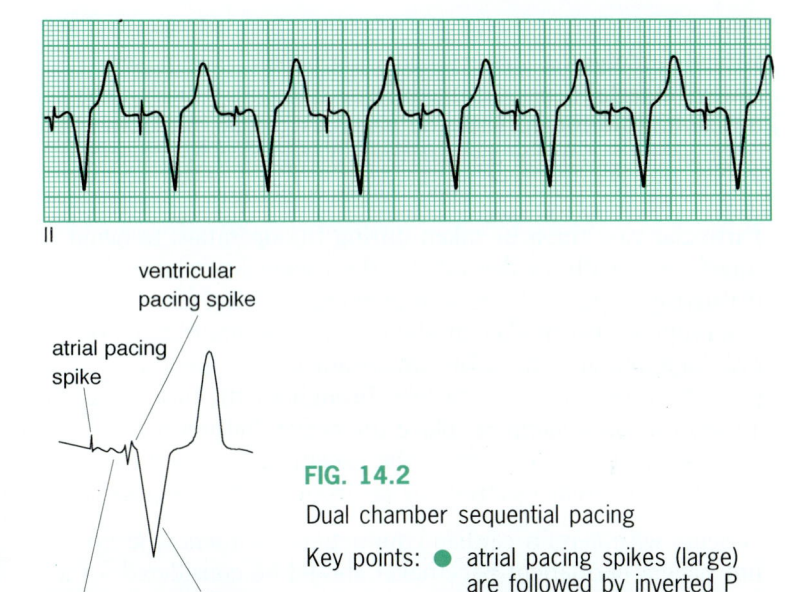

QRS complex. Alternatively, in dual-chamber sequential pacing, the P wave will be followed by a pacing spike from the ventricular lead and a broad QRS complex (Fig. 14.2).

Failure of a pacing spike to be followed by depolarization indicates a problem with 'capture' and a cardiologist should be contacted to arrange a pacemaker check.

PACEMAKERS AND SURGERY

Pacemakers are relevant in surgery for two reasons:

- permanent pacemakers and diathermy
- temporary prophylactic perioperative pacing.

Surgeons and anaesthetists must always be made aware if a patient undergoing surgery has a permanent pacemaker. Always ascertain the pacemaker type (patients usually carry an identification card with the pacemaker code on it) and the original indication for its insertion. It may also be advisable to arrange a check of the pacemaker before and after surgery.

Particular care must be taken during the operation to avoid interference with, or damage to, the pacemaker from diathermy. A particular risk of diathermy is that of inappropriate pacemaker inhibition, causing bradycardia or even asystole; it is therefore important to monitor the patient's ventricular rate closely throughout the procedure. To minimize the dangers, place the active diathermy electrode at least 15 cm from the pacemaker's generator box, and the indifferent electrode as far from the box as possible.

Patients with certain cardiac conduction disorders who do **not** have a permanent pacemaker should be considered for a temporary pacemaker if they are about to undergo general anaesthesia. Temporary pacing is indicated in:

- third-degree AV block
- second-degree AV block.

Pacing is not usually necessary for bifascicular block unless the patient has a history of presyncope or syncope. Consult a cardiologist for further guidance.

15

EXERCISE ECG TESTING

The exercise ECG can be a valuable tool for the assessment of patients with ischaemic heart disease and exercise-related arrhythmias. However, failure to interpret exercise ECGs correctly limits their usefulness.

In this chapter, we will help you to answer the following questions:

- What are the indications for an exercise ECG?
- What are the risks of an exercise ECG?
- How do I perform an exercise ECG?
- When do I stop an exercise ECG?
- How do I interpret an exercise ECG?

WHAT ARE THE INDICATIONS FOR AN EXERCISE ECG?

Exercise ECG testing can be useful in:

- diagnosing chest pain
- risk stratification in stable angina
- risk stratification after myocardial infarction
- assessing exercise-induced arrhythmias
- assessing the need for a permanent pacemaker
- assessing exercise tolerance
- assessing response to treatment.

Exercise ECG testing should always be undertaken with a specific question in mind, and an appreciation of its limitations. In particular, it should only be performed if the information you are likely to gain outweighs the potential (albeit small) risks.

WHAT ARE THE RISKS OF AN EXERCISE ECG?

As with all procedures, exercise ECG testing carries risks:

- a morbidity of 2.4 in 10 000
- a mortality of 1 in 10 000 (within 1 week of testing).

To minimize the risks, always take a patient history and perform an examination to check for **absolute** contraindications to exercise ECG testing (Table 15.1).

Table 15.1 Absolute contraindications to an exercise ECG

- Recent myocardial infarction (within 7 days)
- Unstable angina (rest pain within previous 48 h)
- Severe aortic stenosis or hypertrophic obstructive cardiomyopathy
- Acute myocarditis
- Acute pericarditis
- Uncontrolled hypertension
  - systolic BP over 250 mmHg
  - diastolic BP over 120 mmHg
- Uncontrolled heart failure
- Recent thromboembolic episode (pulmonary or systemic)
- Acute febrile illness

In addition, there are several **relative** contraindications in which an exercise ECG should only be performed with a full awareness of the increased risks involved and under close medical supervision (Table 15.2).

Table 15.2 Relative contraindications to an exercise ECG

- Recent myocardial infarction (within 7 days to 1 month[a])
- Known **severe** coronary artery disease
- Known serious risk of arrhythmia
- Mild or moderate aortic stenosis or hypertrophic obstructive cardiomyopathy
- Pulmonary hypertension
- Significant left ventricular dysfunction
- Aneurysm (ventricular or aortic)
- Highly abnormal resting ECG[b]
  - left or right bundle branch block
  - digoxin effect
- Frail patients

[a]A submaximal exercise test should be used.
[b]An exercise thallium scan can be considered instead.

HOW DO I PERFORM AN EXERCISE ECG?

Unless the exercise test is being performed to assess the effectiveness of therapy, patients should be advised to tail off any existing antianginal treatment over the 3 days before the test. They can use sublingual GTN until 1 h before the test.

On the day of the test, ensure that two people (trained in CPR) are present for supervision and that all the necessary drugs and equipment for CPR are available.

After explaining the test to the patient and checking for contraindications (see previous section), decide which exercise protocol to use. There are many different protocols available, but the two most commonly used are:

- the Bruce protocol
- the modified Bruce protocol.

The modified Bruce protocol begins with a lighter workload than the Bruce protocol, and is particularly suitable for frail patients or those being assessed after a recent myocardial infarction (Fig. 15.1).

EXERCISE PROTOCOL

FIG. 15.1
The Bruce and modified Bruce protocols

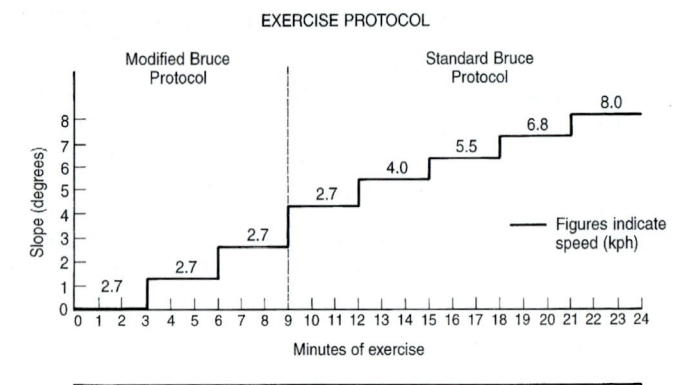

Protocol	Modified Bruce			Standard Bruce				
Stage	01	02	03	1	2	3	4	5
Speed (kph)	2.7	2.7	2.7	2.7	4.0	5.5	6.8	8.0
Slope (degrees)	0	1.3	2.6	4.3	5.4	6.3	7.2	8.1

After reviewing the patient's resting ECG and checking their blood pressure, they can commence exercise. Monitor their symptoms and ECG throughout, and check their blood pressure every 3 min. Reasons for stopping the test are discussed on the following page.

After the completion of exercise, continue to monitor the patient's ECG and blood pressure until any symptoms or ECG changes have fully resolved.

What is a MET?

The workload at each level of an exercise protocol can be expressed in terms of metabolic equivalents (or METs). One MET, the rate of oxygen consumption by a normal person at rest, is 3.5 ml/kg per min. To perform the activities of daily living requires 5 METs.

WHEN DO I STOP AN EXERCISE ECG?

One indicator of a good prognosis is the ability to achieve a target heart rate with no symptoms or significant ECG changes. The target heart rate is calculated thus:
Target heart rate = 220 − patient's age (in years)

However, a number of events may require the exercise test to be stopped before the target heart rate is reached. The test *must* be stopped if:

- the patient asks for the test to be stopped
- the systolic BP falls by >20 mmHg
- the heart rate falls by >10 beats per minute
- sustained ventricular or supraventricular arrhythmias occur.

In addition, you should consider stopping the test if the patient develops:

- >2 mm ST segment depression and chest pain
- >3 mm asymptomatic ST segment depression
- conduction disturbance and chest pain
- non-sustained ventricular tachycardia
- dizziness
- marked or disproportionate breathlessness
- severe fatigue or exhaustion.

HOW DO I INTERPRET AN EXERCISE ECG?

If the indication for the exercise ECG was the induction of an exercise-related arrhythmia, it should be fairly clear whether the test has succeeded in doing so. The interpretation of arrhythmias was the subject of the earlier chapters in this book. Repeating the exercise test once the patient has been established on treatment can be helpful in assessing its efficacy.

Exercise ECGs performed for ischaemic heart disease are often poorly interpreted, and part of the reason for this is a failure to appreciate their limitations. Exercise ECG testing is *not* a 'gold-standard' test for ischaemic heart disease, and so you should be careful about reporting tests in 'black or white' terms such as 'positive' or 'negative'. It may be more useful instead to estimate the *probability* that a patient has coronary artery disease (see below).

The most common indicator of coronary artery disease upon exercise is the development of ST segment depression; and the greater the depression, the higher the probability of coronary artery disease. However, care must be taken when measuring ST segment depression during exercise, as depression of the **J point** (the junction of the S wave and ST segment) is normal. The ST segment upslopes sharply after the J point, and returns to the baseline within 60 ms (1.5 small squares). You must therefore measure ST segment depression **80 ms (2 small squares) beyond the J point** (Fig. 15.2).

ST segment depression is not the only significant result, however. T wave inversion may develop during exercise, as may bundle branch block, although these can occur without

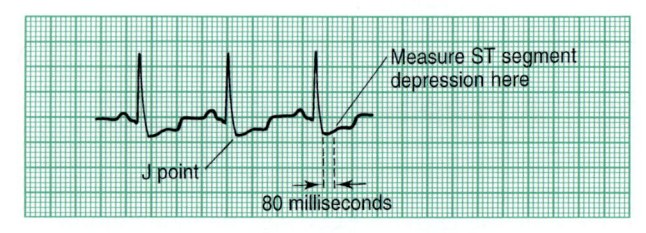

FIG. 15.2

The J point

Key points:
- the J point is the junction of the S wave and ST segment
- measure ST segment depression 80 ms after the J point

significant coronary artery disease. A fall in systolic blood pressure often indicates severe coronary artery disease.

The ECGs in Fig. 15.3 were recorded in a patient with three-vessel coronary artery disease, and show the ST segment changes before, during and after exercise.

The probability of a patient having coronary artery disease depends upon:

- gender (fewer false positives in men)
- age (fewer false positives in older patients)
- degree of ST segment depression
- accompanying symptoms.

Table 15.3 allows you to estimate a patient's probability of coronary artery disease based upon these parameters.

The results of exercise ECG testing also allow for risk stratification by using a nomogram, such as the one in Fig. 15.4, to predict mortality.

234 MAKING SENSE OF THE ECG

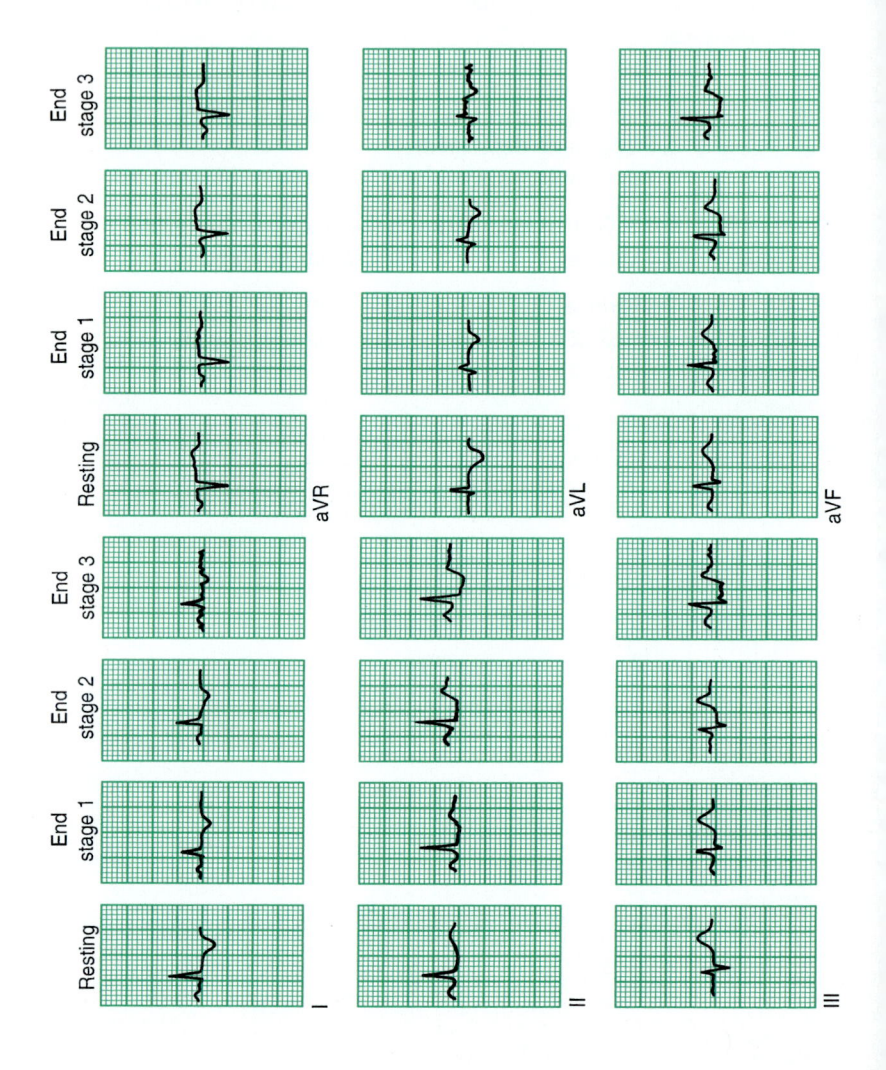

15

FIG. 15.3

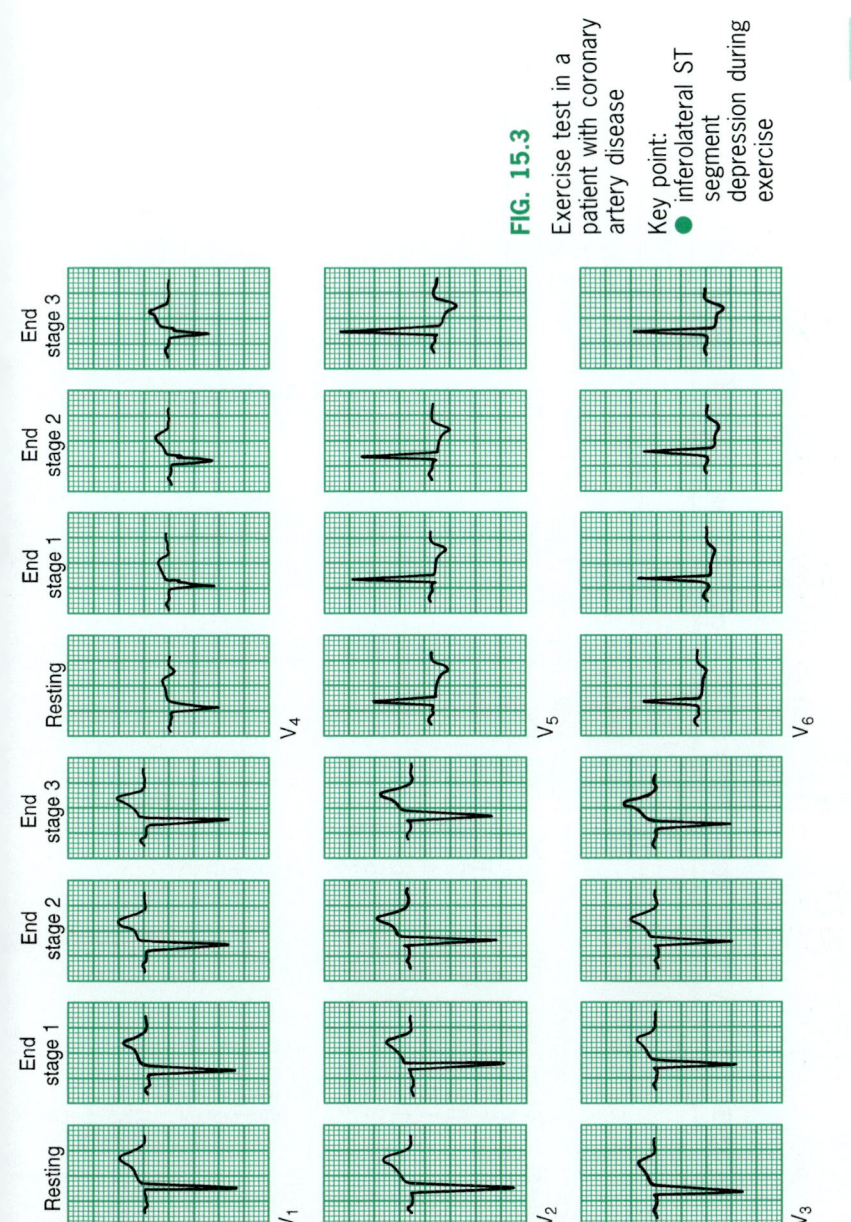

Exercise test in a patient with coronary artery disease

Key point:
- inferolateral ST segment depression during exercise

Table 15.3 Probability (%) of coronary artery disease according to age, sex and exercise test findings

Age (years)	ST segment depression (mm)	Male patients - None	Male - Non-anginal chest pain	Male - Atypical angina	Male - Typical angina	Female - None	Female - Non-anginal chest pain	Female - Atypical angina	Female - Typical angina
30–39	0–0.5	<1	1	6	25	<1	<1	1	7
	0.5–1.0	2	5	21	68	<1	1	4	24
	1.0–1.5	4	10	38	83	1	2	9	42
	1.5–2.0	8	19	55	91	1	3	16	59
	2.0–2.5	18	38	76	96	3	8	33	79
	>2.5	43	68	92	99	11	24	63	93
40–49	0–0.5	1	4	16	61	<1	1	3	22
	0.5–1.0	5	13	44	86	1	3	12	53
	1.0–1.5	11	26	64	94	2	6	25	72
	1.5–2.0	20	41	78	97	4	11	39	84
	2.0–2.5	39	65	91	99	10	24	63	93
	>2.5	69	87	97	>99	28	53	86	98

50–59	0–0.5	2	6	25	73	1	2	10	47
	0.5–1.0	9	20	57	91	3	8	31	78
	1.0–1.5	19	37	75	96	7	16	50	89
	1.5–2.0	31	53	86	98	12	28	67	94
	2.0–2.5	54	75	94	99	27	50	84	98
	>2.5	81	91	98	>99	56	78	95	99
60–69	0–0.5	3	8	32	79	2	5	21	69
	0.5–1.0	11	26	65	94	7	17	52	90
	1.0–1.5	23	45	81	97	15	33	72	95
	1.5–2.0	37	62	90	99	25	49	83	98
	2.0–2.5	61	81	96	>99	47	72	93	99
	>2.5	85	94	99	>99	76	90	98	>99

Adapted from Diamond G. A. and Forrester, J. S. 1979. *N. Engl. J. Med.* **300**, 1350–8. Copyright 1996, Massachusetts Medical Society. All rights reserved.

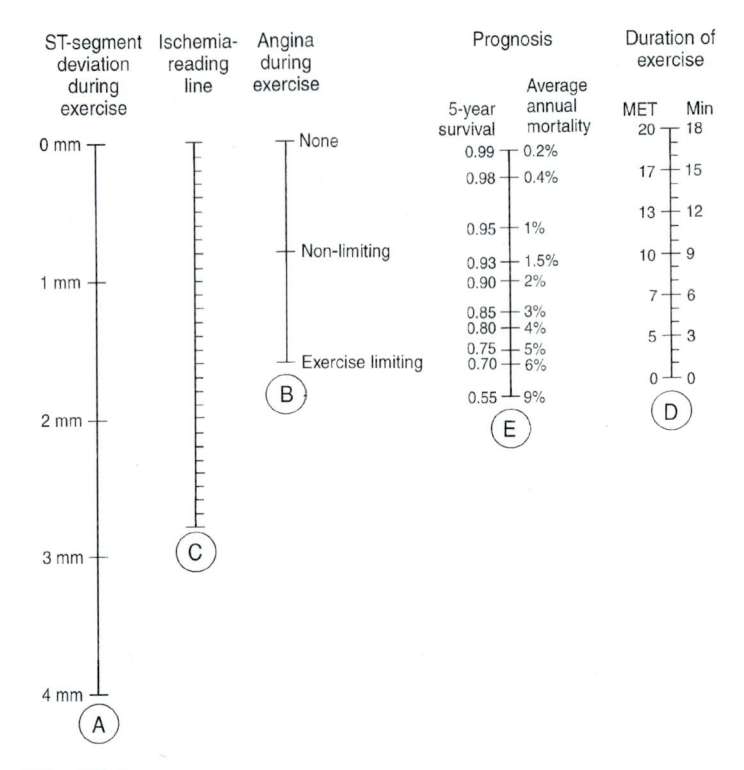

FIG. 15.4

Nomogram for predicting prognosis following exercise testing (Adapted from Mark, D. B. et al. 1991: *N. Engl. J. Med.* **325**, 849–53. Copyright 1996, Massachusetts Medical Society. All rights reserved.)

How to use:

- mark on line A the maximum ST segment deviation seen during exercise
- mark on line B the degree of angina during exercise
- join the marks on lines A and B with a straight line
- mark the point where this line crosses line C (the 'ischaemia-reading line')
- mark on line D the duration of exercise (Bruce protocol) or METs achieved
- join the marks on lines C and D with a straight line
- where this line crosses line E, read off the patient's predicted mortality

16

CARDIOPULMONARY RESUSCITATION

Many cardiac arrests are poorly managed because of disorganization of the cardiac arrest team and a lack of knowledge about recommended procedures by its members. In particular, arrhythmias are frequently incorrectly diagnosed and treated. The rapid identification and treatment of arrhythmias is a cornerstone of successful cardiopulmonary resuscitation (CPR), and for this reason we have included this section on CPR to help you answer the following questions:

- What should I do if a patient collapses?
- How do I perform basic life support?
- How do I perform advanced life support?
- How do I diagnose the arrhythmias?
- When – and how – should I use the defibrillator?
- How do I treat VF and pulseless VT?
- How do I treat asystole?
- How do I treat electromechanical dissociation?
- How do I manage peri-arrest arrhythmias?
- How should I conduct others during the arrest?
- What should I do after the arrest?

The guidelines in this chapter are based upon the 1997 recommendations of the European Resuscitation Council.

Keeping your hands in position, release the pressure and repeat the chest compression at a rate of 100 compressions per minute. The time taken for each chest compression should equal the time taken to release the pressure. Follow every fifteen chest compressions by two ventilations. A cerebral blood flow of at least 20% of normal needs to be maintained for a full neurological recovery.

With two rescuers, it is recommended that one rescuer alternately performs both chest compression and expired air respiration (at a ratio of 5:1), while the second rescuer obtains help. The second rescuer can take over when the first rescuer tires.

Repeat this a total of 10 times. If nobody has heard your call for help, you may quickly stop at this point to find or telephone for assistance. However, return to the patient as soon as you can to continue expired air respiration. Check for spontaneous respiration and a pulse after every 10 breaths.

HOW DO I PERFORM ADVANCED LIFE SUPPORT?

Advanced life support commences as soon as you have access to a defibrillator and suitable drugs. When a full cardiac arrest team is present in hospital, specific tasks can be assigned to individuals (see page 253).

Lose no time in attaching a cardiac monitor to the patient (alternatively, you can monitor the ECG through the defibrillator paddles) and studying the rhythm disorder to make a diagnosis. You must make sure that cardio-pulmonary resuscitation continues until you have decided what the heart rhythm is. Nominate specific individuals to take over basic life support at regular intervals as resuscitation can be very tiring.

HOW DO I DIAGNOSE THE ARRHYTHMIAS?

Remember: time is of the essence. Rapid and correct identification and treatment of cardiac rhythm abnormalities is central to the delivery of effective advanced life support.

You must be able to recognize with confidence each of the four arrhythmias that occur in cardiac arrest:

- ventricular fibrillation
- pulseless ventricular tachycardia
- asystole
- electromechanical dissociation.

In addition, you should know how to manage three arrhythmias that may appear during or shortly after cardiac arrest:

- bradycardia (see Sinus bradycardia page 34)
- narrow complex tachycardia (see How do I distinguish between VT and SVT? page 73)
- broad complex tachycardia (see How do I distinguish between VT and SVT? page 73)

Ventricular Fibrillation

Ventricular fibrillation (VF) is the commonest initial arrhythmia causing cardiac arrest and appears as a chaotic rhythm on the ECG (Figure 16.1). If the monitor is faulty, or the gain turned too low, it can be mistaken for asystole.

Pulseless Ventricular Tachycardia

Ventricular tachycardia (VT) appears as a broad complex rapid cardiac rhythm (Figure 16.2), and can cause haemodynamic collapse (hence 'pulseless').

Asystole

Asystole implies there is no spontaneous electrical cardiac activity, and thus the ECG is simply a flat line (Figure 16.3).

244 MAKING SENSE OF THE ECG

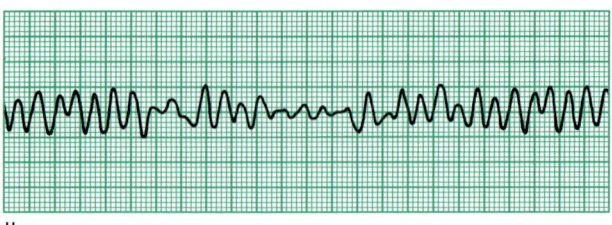

FIG. 16.1

Ventricular fibrillation

Key point: ● chaotic ventricular activity

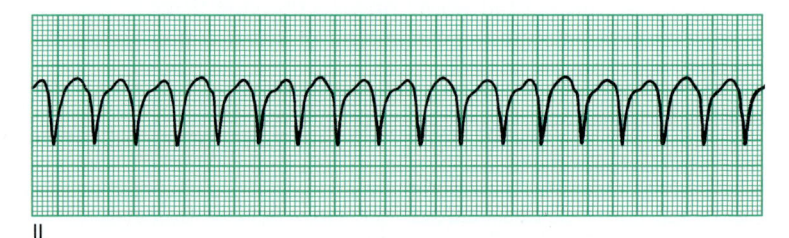

FIG. 16.2

Ventricular tachycardia

Key point: ● broad-complex tachycardia

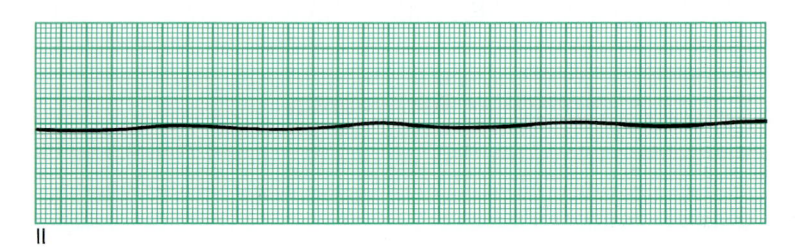

FIG. 16.3

Asystole

Key point: ● 'flat line' (no spontaneous activity)

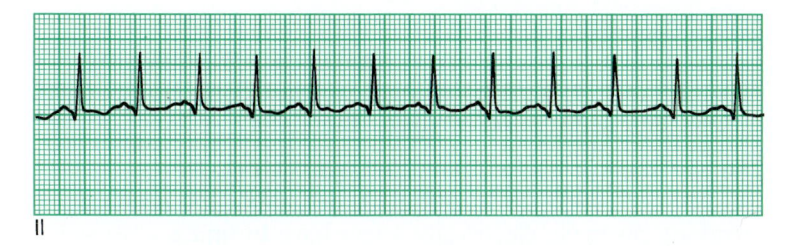

FIG. 16.4

Electromechanical dissociation

Key point: ● QRS complexes in the absence of a cardiac output

Electromechanical dissociation

Electromechanical dissociation (EMD) occurs when the heart continues to work electrically (the ECG continues to show QRS complexes, Figure 16.4), but fails to provide a circulation.

Having confidently diagnosed the rhythm disorder, move on quickly to provide the appropriate treatment.

WHEN – AND HOW – SHOULD I USE THE DEFIBRILLATOR?

Defibrillation is used during a cardiac arrest to convert the heart from an abnormal rhythm to sinus rhythm (or, at least, to a rhythm that restores a cardiac output). Hence, you must use the defibrillator when you have diagnosed:

● ventricular fibrillation
● pulseless ventricular tachycardia.

In addition, you should defibrillate the patient if you think they are in asystole but can't be **entirely** confident that it isn't small complex ('fine') ventricular fibrillation.

However, there is no point in defibrillating a patient if you are **confident** that they are in asystole. Defibrillation just changes one rhythm to another – it will not restart the heart when there is no initial rhythm.

Finally, there is also no point in defibrillating electromechanical dissociation. By definition, the heart is working normally electrically – you have to find a mechanical reason for the lack of a cardiac output.

Ensure you are familiar with the defibrillators used in your workplace, as you cannot afford to waste time should you need to use one. When preparing to defibrillate a patient rapidly check the following:

- all nitrate patches have been removed from the patient (risk of burns);
- the paddles are at least 15 cm from a permanent pacemaker box.

Apply electrode jelly or gel pads to the skin below the paddles, but don't spread jelly between the paddles as this can cause a 'short-circuit'. Note also that some gel pads need replacing between shocks.

After warning everyone to stand clear of the patient and bed, and checking they have done so, proceed to deliver the DC shocks (as described in the appropriate protocol) without delay.

HOW DO I TREAT VF AND PULSELESS VT?

Both arrhythmias are treated identically (Figure 16.5). If a precordial thump has failed to work, electrical defibrillation must be provided as quickly as possible, as described in the previous section. Start with three DC shocks in rapid succession, at energies of 200 J, 200 J and then 360 J. Pause only briefly between shocks to assess the patient's rhythm

CARDIOPULMONARY RESUSCITATION

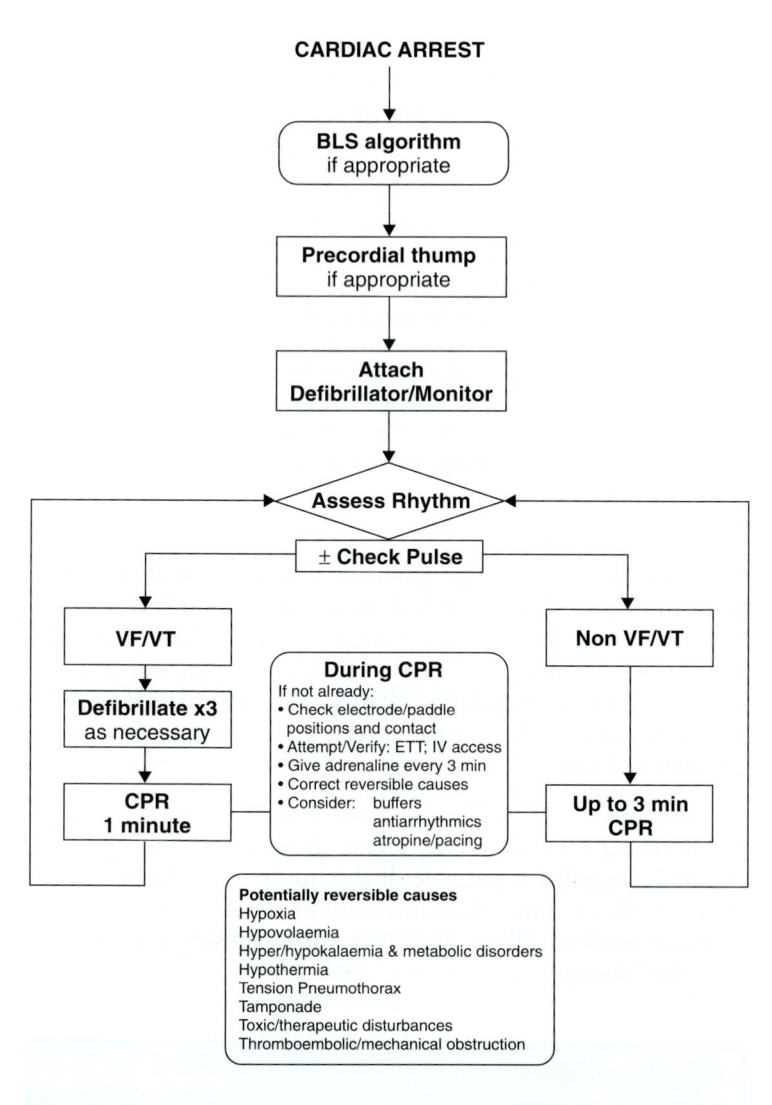

CARDIAC ARREST
↓
BLS algorithm if appropriate
↓
Precordial thump if appropriate
↓
Attach Defibrillator/Monitor
↓
Assess Rhythm
± Check Pulse

VF/VT
↓
Defibrillate x3 as necessary
↓
CPR 1 minute

During CPR
If not already:
- Check electrode/paddle positions and contact
- Attempt/Verify: ETT; IV access
- Give adrenaline every 3 min
- Correct reversible causes
- Consider: buffers
             antiarrhythmics
             atropine/pacing

Non VF/VT
↓
Up to 3 min CPR

Potentially reversible causes
Hypoxia
Hypovolaemia
Hyper/hypokalaemia & metabolic disorders
Hypothermia
Tension Pneumothorax
Tamponade
Toxic/therapeutic disturbances
Thromboembolic/mechanical obstruction

FIG. 16.5

Source: 1997 Resuscitation Guidelines for the United Kingdom. Modified from the ILCOR Advisory Statement. Internet address – http://www.nda.ox.ac.uk/rc-uk/pages/faq.htm#aals

DRUG POINT

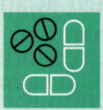

Atropine acts by reducing vagal (parasympathetic) nerve activity on the heart and thereby increases the heart rate, although its value in asystole has not been proven.

After three loops, if the patient is still asystolic, consider pacing if electrical activity (P waves or QRS complexes) becomes evident, using a transvenous pacing wire or transthoracic pacing.

HOW DO I TREAT ELECTROMECHANICAL DISSOCIATION?

If you diagnose electromechanical dissociation (EMD), always look hard for an underlying, remediable, cause (Table 16.1).

Support the patient according to the management algorithm in Figure 16.5 while looking for, and if possible treating, the cause.

After intubating the patient and gaining intravenous access, administer adrenaline 1mg intravenously and continue basic life support for 3 minutes with a chest compression to

Table 16.1 Causes of electromechanical dissociation

- Cardiac tamponade
- Drug overdose
- Electrolyte disturbance
- Hypothermia
- Hypovolaemia
- Pulmonary embolism
- Tension pneumothorax

ventilation ratio of 5:1. Assess the cardiac rhythm and pulse. If electromechanical dissociation persists, give **one** dose of atropine 3 mg intravenously. Repeat the loop, maintaining basic life support and giving further doses of adrenaline every 3 minutes.

Although high-dose adrenaline (5 mg intravenously), alkalizing agents, calcium and pressor agents can be given, there is no firm evidence for their routine use.

HOW DO I MANAGE PERI-ARREST ARRHYTHMIAS?

You must be able to recognize and be prepared to treat promptly any arrhythmia that develops during or shortly after cardiac arrest.

Bradycardia

You should quickly assess the patient's ECG and clinical condition, as these will help you decide the likelihood of the patient deteriorating (Figure 3.3). If there is a risk of asystole, atropine 500 mcg intravenously will usually increase heart rate, but several doses may be needed. Seek expert advice as temporary pacing may be necessary. As a temporary measure, external pacing or intravenous isoprenaline may be started.

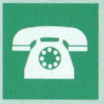

> **SEEK HELP**
>
> Expert help may be needed for patients with a peri-arrest bradycardia where there is a risk of asystole or which does not respond to atropine.

Narrow complex tachycardia

Inhibition of the vagus nerve by the Valsalva manoeuvre or carotid sinus massage may slow and terminate supraventricular tachycardia. Failing this, increasing boluses of adenosine can be given intravenously. If these are ineffective, or if the patient has 'fast' atrial fibrillation, call for expert help.

Quickly assess the patient's clinical signs for evidence of a poor prognosis – if any of these are present, and prepare to sedate the patient for DC cardioversion. With the defibrillator set to *synchronized* mode, give a 100 J shock and re-assess the patient. If the arrhythmia persists, try further shocks of 200 J and 360 J. A bolus of amiodarone followed by an infusion may improve the chances of successful DC cardioversion to sinus rhythm.

If your clinical assessment does not suggest a poor prognosis, start treatment with either esmolol, digoxin, verapamil or amiodarone – all are effective and most hospitals will stock at least two of these drugs. Exceptionally, overdrive pacing may be necessary.

Broad complex tachycardia

Always feel the carotid or other large artery for a pulse – if you cannot feel one, give a precordial thump and follow the VF/pulseless VT protocol (Figure 16.5).

Next carry out a brief clinical assessment. Signs and symptoms which suggest a poor prognosis include low blood pressure, heart failure, very fast heart rate or symptoms of chest pain. You should get expert help quickly and prepare to sedate the patient for DC cardioversion. With the defibrillator set to *synchronized* mode, give a 100 J shock and re-assess the patient. If the arrhythmia persists, try further shocks of 200 J and 360 J. A bolus followed by an infusion of lignocaine or intravenous magnesium can be effective. Low serum levels of potassium should be increased with intravenous potassium chloride. When the infusions have been running for a while, the patient may respond to DC cardioversion, but in exceptional cases it may be necessary to try other anti-arrhythmic drugs or overdrive pacing.

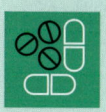

> **DRUG POINT**
>
> It is not necessary to know the serum level before giving intravenous magnesium – it may be effective even when the serum level is normal.

If your clinical assessment does not suggest a poor prognosis, start treatment at once with a bolus and then an infusion of lignocaine, correct serum potassium if this is low and give magnesium intravenously. If the arrhythmia persists, arrange to cardiovert the patient and call for expert help. A bolus of amiodarone followed by an infusion may improve the chances of successful DC cardioversion to sinus rhythm.

HOW SHOULD I CONDUCT OTHERS DURING THE ARREST?

A poorly-trained and inexperienced arrest team will conduct a cardiac arrest in a disorganized manner. It is essential that all members of the team are familiar with basic and advanced life support guidelines and that the most experienced person present takes overall control of the situation.

While diagnosing the arrhythmias and taking decisions accordingly, the team leader must direct others with clear instructions to specified individuals. Ideally, there should be one member of the team for each of the following tasks:

- chest compression (swapping with others when tired)
- defibrillation
- ventilating and/or intubating the patient

- obtaining intravenous access
- drawing up the necessary drugs
- keeping a record of events, and counting the seconds out loud whenever CPR is interrupted

The team leader should also discuss with the rest of the team when further resuscitation appears futile and, if the others are in agreement, terminate resuscitation efforts.

WHAT SHOULD I DO AFTER THE ARREST?

Following a successful resuscitation the patient will need observation and monitoring, ideally on an intensive or coronary care unit. Particularly important is the management of the patient's airway and breathing, especially if their conscious level is reduced, and artificial ventilation may be needed.

You will need to check:

- blood urea and electrolytes
- 12-lead ECG
- chest X-ray

in addition to monitoring or regularly checking:

- vital signs
- urine output
- ECG monitoring
- arterial blood gases and acid-base balance

Finally, do not forget the patient's relatives. Speak to them as soon as possible after the arrest.

FURTHER READING

ECG interpretation

Conover, M. B. 1996: *Understanding electrocardiography*, 7th edn. St Louis, MO: Mosby. ISBN 0-8151-1927-5.
Hampton, J. R. 1992: *The ECG made easy*, 4th edn. Edinburgh: Churchill Livingstone. ISBN 0-443-04507-0.
Hampton, J. R. 1992: *The ECG in practice*, 2nd edn. Edinburgh: Churchill Livingstone. ISBN 0-443-04506-2.

Cardiology textbooks

Julian, D. G., Camm, A. J., Fox, K. M., Hull, R. J. C. and Poole-Wilson, P. A. 1996: *Diseases of the heart*, 2nd edn. London: Saunders. ISBN 0-7020-1756-6.
Leatham, A., Bull, C. and Braimbridge, M. V. 1991: *Lecture notes on cardiology*, 3rd edn. Oxford: Blackwell Scientific Publications. ISBN 0-632-01944-1.

CPR guidelines

The 1997 Resuscitation Guidelines for use in the United Kingdom. Resuscitation Council (UK). Resuscitation Council (UK) Publications. These guidelines can be found on the Resuscitation Council (UK) world-wide web site at: http://www.nda.ox.ac.uk/rc-uk/pages/guidelns.htm:

HELP WITH THE NEXT EDITION

We would like to know what you would like to see included (or omitted!) from the next edition of *Making Sense of the ECG*. Please write with your comments or suggestions to:

Dr Andrew R. Houghton
Making Sense of the ECG
c/o Arnold (Publishers)
338 Euston Road
London   NW1 3BH

We will include acknowledgements to all those whose suggestions are used in the next edition.

INDEX

AAI pacemakers 223
ABC, basic life support 240
Absolute contraindications,
    exercise ECG 228
Accelerated idioventricular rhythm
    57
Accessory pathways 49–50, 112,
    139
Address for author 257
Adenosine, for AV re-entry
    tachycardia 54
Adrenaline
    asystole 249
    electromechanical dissociation
        250
    ventricular fibrillation 248
Aide-memoire, bundle branch
    block 147
Airway 241
Alkalizing agents 249
Alternans, electrical 142, 143
Ambulatory ECG recording 40
Amiodarone, atrial fibrillation 48
Amplitude *see* Voltage
Anaesthetics
    pacemakers 226
    Wolff–Parkinson–White
        syndrome 113

Aneurysm
    left ventricle 165–166
Angina
    Prinzmetal's 166–168
    stable 171–173
    unstable 173
Angiotensin-converting enzyme
    inhibitor, myocardial
    infarction 164
Anterior hemiblock, left 89–91
Anterior myocardial infarction
    160, 161
    Mobitz type I AV block 118
    temporary pacing 220
    third-degree AV block 122
Anterolateral myocardial infarction
    160
    right axis deviation 94–95
Anteroseptal myocardial infarction
    160
Antiarrhythmic drugs
    bradycardia in atrial fibrillation
        25
    on QT interval 203
    ventricular fibrillation 248
Antibody, digoxin-specific 175
Anticoagulation, atrial fibrillation
    46–47

260 INDEX

Anti-inflammatory agents,
 pericarditis 169–170
Aortic dissection 159
Arrest team 253–254
Arrhythmias 31–76
 diagnosing 66–75
 cardiopulmonary
  resuscitation 243–245
Artefacts 213–218
Aspartate transaminase 158–159
Aspirin 164, 172
Asystole 25, 243
 management 249–250
Athletes 35
Atrial depolarization 9–10, 69
 abnormal 104
Atrial ectopics 63, 111
Atrial enlargement
 left 106
 right 105–106
Atrial fibrillation 44–48
 absent P waves 99
 bradycardia from
  antiarrhythmics 25
 Wolff–Parkinson–White
  syndrome 54
Atrial flutter 42–44
 P waves 101
Atrial pacing 224
Atrial rate 23
Atrial rhythms 76
Atrial tachycardia 40–42
Atrioventricular node *see* AV
 node
Atrioventricular rhythms 76
Atropine 26
 asystole 250
Author, address for 257
Automatic implantable
 cardiovertor defibrillators
 (AICD) 57

AV block 24, 60, 70, 71
 atrial flutter 42
 atrial tachycardia 41
 first-degree 60, 90, 115–116
 Mobitz type I 117–118
 Mobitz type II 117, 119–120
 pacing 222, 226
 second-degree 24, 60
 third-degree 24, 60, 90,
  117–118, 121–122
 2:1 117, 120
AV dissociation 70, 71, 122
AV junctional ectopics 64
AV junctional escape rhythms 62
AV junctional pacemaker
 (intrinsic) 61, 110
AV junctional rhythms 69
 P wave inversion 104
 PR interval 110–111
AV junctional tachycardia
 100–101
AV nodal re-entry tachycardia
 51–52
AV node 10
 depolarization 20
 sick sinus syndrome 39
AV re-entry tachycardias 48–54
 nodal 51–52
aVR lead, P wave 10
Axis, cardiac 77–96

Baseline 155
Basic life support 240–242
Bazett's formula 197
Beck's triad 141
Beta blockers
 interaction with verapamil 42, 46
 myocardial infarction 164
 Prinzmetal's angina 168
 and tachycardia 36
Bicarbonate 249

INDEX

Bifascicular block 89–91
  pacing 222
Bifid P wave 106–107
Bigeminy 64
Bisphosphonates 199
Black people, T wave inversion 186, 187
Bradycardia 23, 24–26, 30
  see also specific types
Breathing 241
Broad-complex rhythms 68
Broad-complex tachycardias 27–28, 73–75
Bruce protocol 229–230
Bundle branch block 60–61, 144–151
  AV re-entry tachycardia 52
  in bifascicular and trifascicular block 89–90
  exercise ECG 229, 232
  incomplete 151–152
  left 144, 145–146, 149–151, 157
  right 144–151
Bundle branches 12, 13
  left 14
Bundle of His 11
Bundle of James 114–115
Bundle of Kent 112, 139

Caffeine 28
Calcium, intravenous 201
Calibration 19
  incorrect 215–216
Capture beats 73, 75
Cardiac arrest team 253–254
Cardiac axis 77–96
Cardiac enzymes 158–159
Cardiac massage (chest compression) 241–242
Cardiac output, atrial contribution 45

Cardiac tamponade 141–143
Cardiopulmonary resuscitation 239–254
Cardioversion
  DC, atrial fibrillation 47
  medical 56–57
  see also Defibrillation
Carotid sinus massage 43, 44
  for AV re-entry tachycardia 53
Carotid sinus syndrome, pacing 222
Cerebral blood flow 242
Chest compression 241–242
Chest electrodes, placing 18–19
Chest leads 5
  QRS complexes 16
  right-sided 163
Chvostek's sign 201
Complete heart block *see* Third-degree AV block
Conduction disturbances 60–61
Congenital long QT syndromes 59, 205
Contraindications, exercise ECG 228–229
Coronary artery disease
  exercise ECG diagnosis 232, 234–235
  probability figures 236–237
  see also Angina; Myocardial infarction
Coronary artery spasm 166–168
Corrected QT interval 196–197
Corticosteroids, pericarditis 170
Cosine (trigonometrical) 87
Creatine kinase 158–159

DC cardioversion, atrial fibrillation 47
DDD pacemakers 223

Defibrillation
  asystole 249
  cardiopulmonary resuscitation 245–246
  DC cardioversion 47
Delta wave 112, 113
  AV re-entry tachycardia 49, 51
Depolarization 2
Dextrocardia 139–140
  right axis deviation 95
Diathermy, pacemakers 226
Digoxin 174–175
  atrial fibrillation 48
    Wolff–Parkinson–White syndrome 54
  QT interval 200
  toxicity 41, 174–175
  T wave inversion 192, 193
Disodium pamidronate 199
Dissection, aortic 159
Domiciliary ECG 215
Drugs
  for angina 172
  for atrial fibrillation 48
  for atrial flutter 43–44
  endotracheal tube route 248
  first-degree AV block from 115
  negatively chronotropic 25, 71
  positively chronotropic 28
  sinus tachycardia from 36
  tailing off for exercise ECG 229
  for unstable angina 173
  see also Antiarrhythmic drugs
Dual AV nodal pathway 49, 51
Dual-chamber sequential pacing 225

Early repolarization (ST segment) 170–171
ECG made easy (J.R. Hampton) xvi, 1

Ectopic beats 63–66, 71
  atrial 63, 111
  AV junctional 64
  ventricular 64–66, 104
Elderly patients, and warfarin 47
Electrical alternans 142, 143
Electrical interference 215
Electrocardiography, recording 17–19
Electrodes 3
  misplacement 213–214
  placing 18–19
Electromechanical dissociation (EMD) 245
  management 250–251
Emphysema 141
Endotracheal tube, drugs via 246
Equipolar deflection 7, 15
Escape rhythms 25, 35, 61–63
Europe, paper speed 216
Exercise ECG 227–238
  contraindications 228–229
  indications 227–228
  interpretation 231–238
  muscle activity 217
  when to stop 231
Expired air respiration 241
External cardiac massage (chest compression) 241–242
External electrical interference 215
Extrasystoles *see* Ectopic beats

'f' waves (fibrillation waves) 44, 99
Fascicular block 152–153
  see also Bifascicular block; Trifascicular block
Fibrillation waves 44, 99
First-degree AV block 60, 90, 115–116

Fluid therapy
  hypercalcaemia 199
  right ventricular infarction 164
Friction rub 169
Frusemide, for hypercalcaemia 199
Full thickness infarct (term) 189
Fusion beats, ventricular
  tachycardia 73, 74

Gain *see* Calibration
Ganong, W.F. *see*
  Lown–Ganong–Levine
  syndrome
Glyceryl trinitrate
  patches and defibrillation 246
  tailing off for exercise ECG 229

Hampton, J.R., *ECG made easy*
  xvi, 1
Heart block *see* AV block
  complete *see* Third-degree AV
  block
Heart failure, right sided 164
Heart rate 21–30
  target for exercise ECG 231
Hemiblock
  left anterior 89–91
  left posterior 95
Hereditary syndromes, long QT
  interval 59, 205
High take-off ST segment
  170–171
High-dose adrenaline 250
His, bundle of 11
Holter monitoring 40
Home ECG 215
Hyperacute T wave 156, 157, 168
Hypercalcaemia 198–200, 210
  U wave 199, 210
Hyperkalaemia 181–182
  absent P waves 100

Hyperthermia 198
Hyperthyroidism 210
Hypertrophy *see* Ventricular
  hypertrophy
Hypocalcaemia 201–203
Hypokalaemia 184–185, 209–210
  and digoxin 175
Hypotension, right ventricular
  infarction 164
Hypothyroidism 186

Incomplete bundle branch block
  151–152
Independent P wave activity 73,
  74, 101–102
Inferior myocardial infarction 6–8,
  160, 161, 162
  left axis deviation 92–93
  Mobitz type I AV block 118
  temporary pacing 220
  third-degree AV block 121–122
Inferolateral myocardial infarction
  160
Intensive care, after cardiac arrest
  254
Intravenous access,
  cardiopulmonary
  resuscitation 248
Intravenous fluid therapy
  hypercalcaemia 199
  right ventricular infarction 164
Introductory textbook xvi, 1
Irregular rhythm 71
Irregularly irregular rhythm 45
Isoelectric QRS complex 81
Isoprenaline 26

J point 232
James, bundle of 114–115
Jervell and Lange-Nielsen
  syndrome 205

Kartagener's syndrome 140
Kent, bundle of 112, 139
'Kiss of life' (expired air respiration) 241

Lactate dehydrogenase 158–159
Lateral myocardial infarction 8, 160
Leads 3–8
Left anterior hemiblock 89–91
Left atrial enlargement 106
Left axis deviation 85, 89–93, 96
Left bundle branch 14
   block 144, 145–146, 149–151, 157
Left posterior hemiblock 95
Left ventricular aneurysm 165–166
Left ventricular hypertrophy 131, 135, 192
Life support, advanced *vs* basic 240
Limb electrodes
   misplaced 213–214
   placing 18–19
Limb leads 4, 80
Long QT syndromes 59, 205
Lown–Ganong–Levine syndrome 114–115
Lyme disease 122

Malignant vasovagal syndrome, pacing 222
Measurement
   cardiac axis 81–88
   heart rate 21–23
   time duration 3
   voltage 3
Metabolic equivalents (METs) 230
Mnemonic, bundle branch block 147
Mobitz type I AV block 117–118

Mobitz type II AV block 117, 119–120
Modified Bruce protocol 229–230
Monitoring
   after cardiac arrest 254
   cardiopulmonary resuscitation 242
Morbidity, exercise ECG 228
'Morrow' 147
Mortality, exercise ECG 228
Mouth-to-mouth respiration 241
Muscles, tension 2, 217
Myocardial infarction 156–165
   Mobitz type I AV block 118
   Q wave 128–131 *see also* Q wave myocardial infarction
   ST elevation 156–164
   T waves 156, 157, 182–183
   inversion 188–191
   temporary pacing 220
   see also specific sites e.g. Anterior, Inferior
Myocardial ischaemia 171–173
   T wave inversion 188
Myocarditis 203–204

Narrow-complex rhythms 68
Narrow-complex tachycardias 27
Negative QRS complexes 13–16
   axis measurement 83–86
Negatively chronotropic drugs 25, 71
Nitrate *see* Glyceryl trinitrate
Nomogram, exercise ECG 233, 238
Non-Q wave myocardial infarction 188–191
Normal cardiac axis 77, 83–85
Normal ECG
   QRS complex 133
   T wave inversion 186

Obesity 89, 141
Overdrive pacing 220–221
Oxygen consumption rates 230

P mitrale 106–107
P pulmonale 105–106
P wave 2, 20, 97–108
  arrhythmia diagnosis 69
  atrial ectopics 63
  atrial rate 23
  atrial tachycardia 41
  AV junctional ectopics 64
  AV re-entry tachycardia 52
  axis 88
  inversion 102–104
  mechanism 9
  missing 98–102
  orientation 6, 7
  sinoatrial block 60
  tall 105–106
  ventricular tachycardia 73, 74, 101–102, 104
  wide 106–107
Pacemakers (artificial) 219–226
  see also Permanent and Temporary pacemakers
Pacemakers (subsidiary) 61, 110
Pacing, asystole 250
Pacing spikes 224–225
Pain
  aortic dissection 159
  myocardial infarction 158
  pericarditis 169
Palpitations, history-taking 28
Pamidronate, disodium 199
Paper speed 3, 19, 21
  incorrect 216
Paroxysmal atrial fibrillation 48
Paroxysmal tachycardia, sick sinus syndrome 24, 39, 40

Partial bundle branch block 151–152
Patient movement 216–217
Pericardial effusion 141–143, 186
Pericarditis 169–170
Permanent pacemakers 219, 221–223
  and defibrillation 246
  for sick sinus syndrome 40
Positive QRS complexes 13–16
  axis measurement 81–86
Positively chronotropic drugs 28
Posterior hemiblock, left 95
Posterior myocardial infarction 173
  QRS complex 138–139
  T waves 182–183
PR interval 11, 20, 109–123
  long 115–116
  short 110–115
Precordial thump 240
Pregnancy 89
Premature beats *see* Ectopic beats
Primary ventricular fibrillation 59
Prinzmetal's angina 166–168
Pseudonormalization, T wave 188
Pulmonary embolism 36, 128
Pulseless ventricular tachycardia 243
  management 246–249
Pulsus paradoxus 141–142
Purkinje fibres 13

Q wave 2, 11, 125–132
  septal 147
Q wave myocardial infarction 156–165, 188–191
QRS complex 11–16, 20, 133–154
  abnormal shape 151–153
  AV re-entry tachycardia 52
  axis measurement 81–88

QRS complex *continued*
  small 140–143
  tachycardia 27–29
  ventricular ectopics 64
  ventricular rhythms 68
  wide 143–151
QT interval 16, 20, 195–206
  long 59, 200–205, 206
  short 197–200, 206
Quinidine 175

'R on T' ectopics 64
R wave 2, 11, 15
  'dominant' 136, 138
  size 134
R wave 144, 147
Rate *see* Heart rate
Rate responsive pacemakers 223–224
Recording, electrocardiography 17–19
Recurrent (secondary) ventricular fibrillation 59
Re-entry tachycardias *see* AV re-entry tachycardias
Reference point, cardiac axis 79
Relative contraindications, exercise ECG 228–229
Repolarization 2, 16
  early (ST segment) 170–171
Resistant atrial fibrillation 48
Respiration
  basic life support 240–242
  sinus arrhythmia 37–38
Retrograde conduction 49, 101
'Reverse tick' ST segment 174, 175
Rheumatoid carditis 203
Rhythm strip 31
Right atrial enlargement 105–106
Right axis deviation 85, 93–95, 96

Right bundle branch block 144–151
Right ventricle, myocardial infarction 163–164
Right ventricular hypertrophy 93, 136–137, 192
Right-sided chest leads 163
Romano–Ward syndrome 205
RR interval 197

S wave 2, 13, 15
  size 134
SA node *see* Sinoatrial node
Saddle-shaped ST segments 169
Saline, for hypercalcaemia 199
Sawtooth baseline 43
Secondary ventricular fibrillation 59
Second-degree AV block 24
  pacing 222, 226
Septal depolarization 12, 127, 131
  left bundle branch block 144
Septal Q wave 147
Sick sinus syndrome 24, 38–40
  pacing 222
Signal-averaged ECG 217–218
Sine 87
Sinoatrial block 24, 39, 60, 99–100, 102
Sinoatrial node 9
  depolarization 20
  rhythms 76
Sinus arrest 38, 99–100, 102
Sinus arrhythmia 37–38, 98
Sinus bradycardia 24, 25, 34–35
Sinus rhythm 32–34
Sinus tachycardia 35–37
  P waves 101
Sodium bicarbonate 249
Spikes, pacing 224

S₁Q₁₁₁T₁₁₁ pattern 128
Squares, ECG paper 21–22
ST segment 16, 20, 155–178
   depression 171–176, 178
      exercise ECG 232
   elevation 156–171, 178
   high take-off 170–171
   hyperkalaemia 181
Stable angina 171–173
Steroids, pericarditis 170
'Strain' 135, 136–137
   with ventricular hypertrophy 176, 177, 192
Stroke risk, atrial fibrillation 46
Subendocardial infarct (term) 189
Subsidiary pacemakers 61, 110
Supraventricular rhythms 67–68
Supraventricular tachycardia 75
   bundle branch block 61, 150
   vs ventricular tachycardia 73–75
Surgery
   pacemakers 225–226
   Wolff–Parkinson–White syndrome 113
Sympathetic nervous system, stimulation 35–36
Syncope, and bifascicular block 90–91

T wave 2, 16, 20, 179–194
   axis 88
   inversion 186–191, 194
      exercise ECG 232
   myocardial infarction 156, 157, 182–183, 188–191
   Prinzmetal's angina 168
   small 184–186, 194
   tall 179–183, 194
Tachycardia–bradycardia 39

Tachycardias 23, 27–29, 30
   P waves 100–101
   pacing 220–221
   see also specific types
Tamponade, cardiac 141–143
Tangent (trigonometrical) 87
Target heart rate, for exercise ECG 231
Team leader, cardiac arrest 253–254
Temporary pacemakers 219–221
   for surgery 225–226
   third-degree AV block 122
Tension, muscles 2, 217
Tented T wave 181
Textbook, introductory xvi, 1
Third-degree AV block 24, 60, 90, 117, 121–122
   pacing 222, 226
Thromboembolism, risk factors 47
Thrombolysis
   myocardial infarction 164
   and pacing 221
Time, measurement 4
Timolol 164
Torsades de pointes 57–59, 203, 205
Trifascicular block 90
   pacing 222
Trigonometry 87
Trousseau's sign 201
12-lead ECG 4
24-hour ambulatory ECG recording 40
2:1 AV block 117, 120

U wave 2, 17, 20, 207–211
   hypercalcaemia 199, 210
   hypokalaemia 184–185
   mistaking for T wave 196
Unstable angina 173

Valsalva manoeuvre 52, 54
Vasospastic angina 166–168
Vasovagal syndrome, malignant, pacing 222
Vectors 86
Ventricular ectopics 64
  P wave inversion 104
Ventricular escape rhythms 62
Ventricular fibrillation 28, 55, 59, 243
  management 246–249
Ventricular hypertrophy
  with 'strain' 176, 177, 192
  see also Left and Right ventricular hypertrophy
Ventricular pacemakers (intrinsic) 61
Ventricular rate 21, 23
  atrial flutter 42–43
Ventricular rhythms 67–68, 76, 151
Ventricular tachycardia 55–59
  vs AV re-entry tachycardia 52
  and left axis deviation 93
  P waves 73, 74, 101, 104
  pulseless 243
  management 246–249
  vs supraventricular tachycardia 73–75
Verapamil
  for AV re-entry tachycardia 54
  interaction with beta blockers 42, 46
Voltage, wave size 3
VVI pacemakers 223

Warfarin, atrial fibrillation 46–47
Wenckebach phenomenon (Mobitz type I AV block) 117–118
'William Morrow' 147
Wolff–Parkinson–White syndrome 111–114
  atrial fibrillation 54
  AV re-entry tachycardia 49–50
  left axis deviation 92
  PR interval 111–113
  QRS complex 139, 153
  right axis deviation 94

Zero point, cardiac axis 79